Girl,
Eat That
Burger

Secret Cheat Code to Beat Obesity forever

D.K.R.G.

Girl, Eat That Burger

This Book Belongs To:

____

Girl, Eat That Burger

Girl, Eat That Burger

Secret Cheat Code to Beat Obesity forever

D.K.R.G.

Dishing It Out, get it?
Some Simple things About Me.

Welcome to my world of dieting, where the struggle to lose weight meets the joy of eating everything in sight! Imagine being a full-time food fanatic with an appetite bigger than a buffet line. Honey, I eat when I'm happy, I eat when I'm sad, hell, I'll eat when I'm already full; dessert anyone? It's my kryptonite!

But amidst the endless food cravings and temptation, I've discovered a secret sauce to tame my voracious appetite and keep the scale in check. And guess what? It actually works! I've shared my secrets with friends, and they've been amazed at their results as well.

And Chile, I'm not just your average G.I. Jane trying to shed a few pounds. (Even though sometimes I feel like I'm going to war.) By day, I'm a savvy business owner hustling to make dreams come true. But when I'm not crushing it behind double monitors, I'm a devoted mom to two rambunctious boys and a loving
wife balancing the chaos of family life. With my days packed to the brim, I needed a diet plan as quick and efficient as I am.

That's why I've poured my heart and soul into creating this book and I've included a recipe book filled with 31 quick, high metabolism recipes. These babies are the real deal—easy to whip up in a flash and guaranteed to keep you feeling energized and satisfied throughout the day. And let me tell you, they've been a game-changer for me, my family and friends!

So, consider me your accountability partner on this rollercoaster ride of a lifestyle change with temptations of culinary delights along the way. Together, we'll bid farewell to the old habits—like eating everything in sight—and welcome in a new, healthier version of ourselves. So out with the old and in with the new… you. It's a journey filled with laughter, cravings, and maybe even a few food-related fiascos along the way. But hey, that's all part of the adventure, right?

Now, Girl, grab your seatbelt and hold on tight 'cause we're diving headfirst into this crazy adventure of kicking obesity forever! And, there's no way we're skippin' out on dessert! "Ain't nobody got time foe dat!" (In Sweet Brown voice) But life is too short to let obesity weigh us down. So, let's dig in, laugh loud, and conquer this journey together, sis! This is not Your journey. It's Ours. ♥

Girl, Eat That Burger

Secret Cheat Code to Beat Obesity forever

So many blessing and special thanks to GOD for allowing me full focus for completion of this book.

Thank you to my husband for always supporting me and my two boys for always encouraging me.

D.K.R.G.

TABLE OF CONTENTS

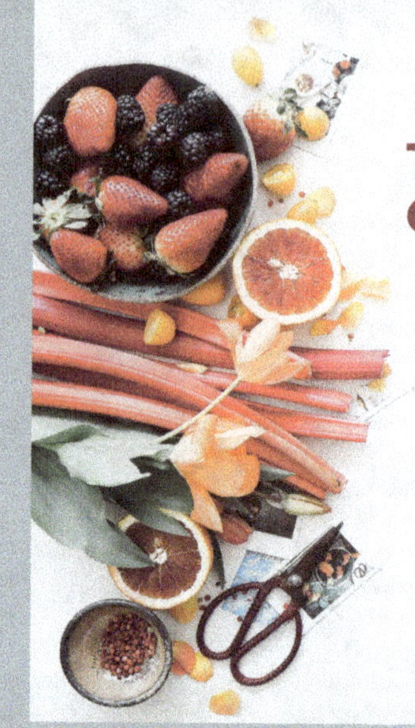

BYE BYE BIG BACK

Burgers for days

Cheat Sheet

Bye Bye Big Back

Table of Contents

Bye Bye Big Back

Table of Contents

Bye Bye Big Back

Table of Contents

Hey Girl, Heyyyy!. If you've stumbled upon this book, chances are you're interested in unbigging your back. Maybe you've tried every fad diet under the sun, from the grapefruit diet to the cabbage soup diet to the "just eat cookies all day" diet (hey, I won't judge). Especially because I once tried the military diet. I was hangry, I was miserable at the same damn time. (In my Future voice). I gained all 3 lbs back the same day I was able to eat again. Let me tell you I will never do it again. We are still not judging, right? Here's the thing: none of those diets are sustainable. Sure, you might lose a few pounds at first, but eventually, you'll end up right back where you started (or even worse, with a bigger back than the one you were just trying to unbig).

That's why I'm not here to talk about diets. Nope, I'm here to talk about lifestyle changes. You see, losing weight isn't just about dropping a few pounds and calling it a day. It's about making sustainable changes to your daily routine that will help you maintain a healthy weight for the years to come.

Now, I know what you're thinking: "But I love tacos too much to give it up!" (Trust me, I feel you.) But here's the thing: you don't have to give up the foods you love. In fact, it's important to indulge every now and then to avoid feeling deprived. But it's all about balance. Maybe you have a slice of pizza for dinner one night, but then you make sure to have a salad with lean protein for lunch the next day. It's all about finding a balance that works for you.

And let's be real, there are some perks to losing weight that go beyond just looking good in a bikini (although that's definitely a plus). For one thing, you'll have more energy to do the things you love. And for another thing, you'll save money on buying new clothes every time your weight fluctuates (seriously, clothes are expensive these days and have you checked your shopping cart lately)?

So, whether you're here because you're tired of crash diets or because you just want to feel better in your own skin, welcome. I'm glad you're here, and excited to embark on this journey together. Who knows, maybe we'll even have some fun along the way (and not just because we'll be able to wear those crop tops and fit into those skinny jeans again).

INTRODUCTION

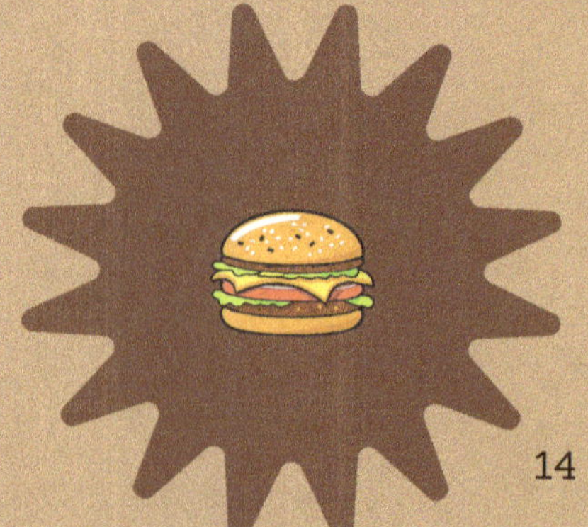

Chapter 1

The Real Culprits Behind Your Weight Gain

Excuses, Excuses, Excuses

Hey Twin, Are you craving a bag of chips like me? First, you start off with a small bag of chips, and before you know it, you've eaten the whole family-size bag. But have you ever stopped to think about why you can't seem to stop yourself from overeating? Well friend, it's time to address the real culprits behind your weight gain.

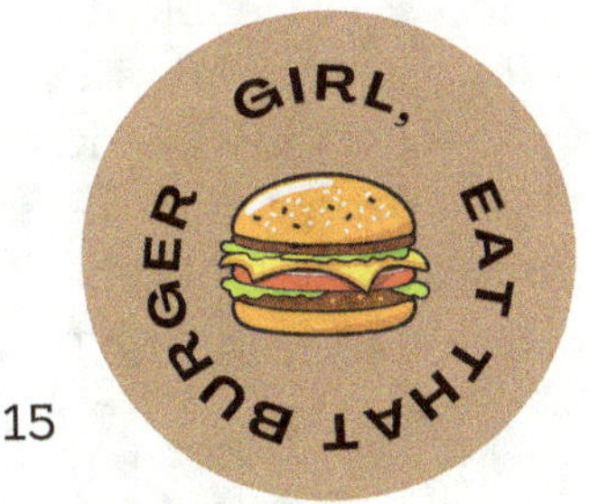

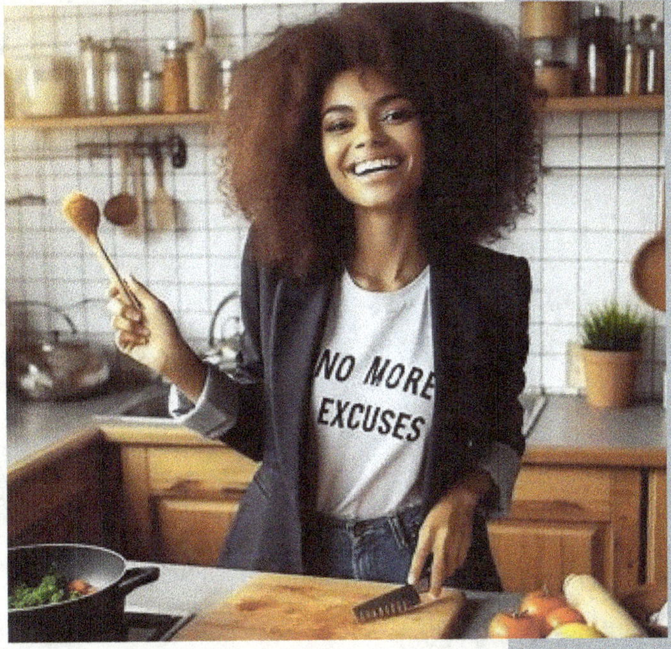

I The "I'm Saving It for Later" Mentality. Do you ever find yourself eating a huge meal because you're afraid you won't have access to the food later? Or maybe you eat the whole bag of chips because you don't want to waste them? Newsflash: you're not a squirrel. You don't need to hoard food in case of a food apocalypse. Unless you're reading this in 2024 and groceries cost an arm and a leg. In which we should all be skinny. However, if you're hungry later, you can always eat again. Make sure it's a small portion.

II The "I'm Bored" Excuse. You know what's not a good reason to eat? Because you're bored. Trust me, that bag of chips is not going to magically entertain you. It's not going to breakdance or hit the Nay Nay. Find yourself a hobby, call a friend, turn on your favorite song and dance your ass off. Do anything else besides eating out of boredom which in return will leave you feeling guilty and bloated.

III The "I Deserve It" Justification. We've all used this excuse before – "I had a tough day, I just want to go home and eat this pint of ice cream." But here's the thing, you deserve to feel good about yourself, not guilty for overindulging. Instead of turning to food for comfort, find healthier options to cope with stress, like exercising or getting a massage.

IV The "I'm Too Tired to Cook" Cop-Out. Yes, cooking can be tiring, but that's not an excuse to order takeout every night. Not only is it expensive, but it's also usually packed with extra calories and sodium. Try meal prepping on the weekends or finding simple, healthy recipes that don't require a lot of effort. And besides, who wants to spend their entire paycheck on greasy foods? Me I do! But that's beside the point. We are holding each other accountable from this point forward.

V The "I Don't Want to Waste It" Rationalization You know what's worse than wasting food? Wasting your health. Just because there's leftover pizza in the fridge doesn't mean you have to eat it. Make a conscious decision to prioritize your health over avoiding food waste.

Chapter II

Eating the Wrong Foods the Right Way

Without the Guilt

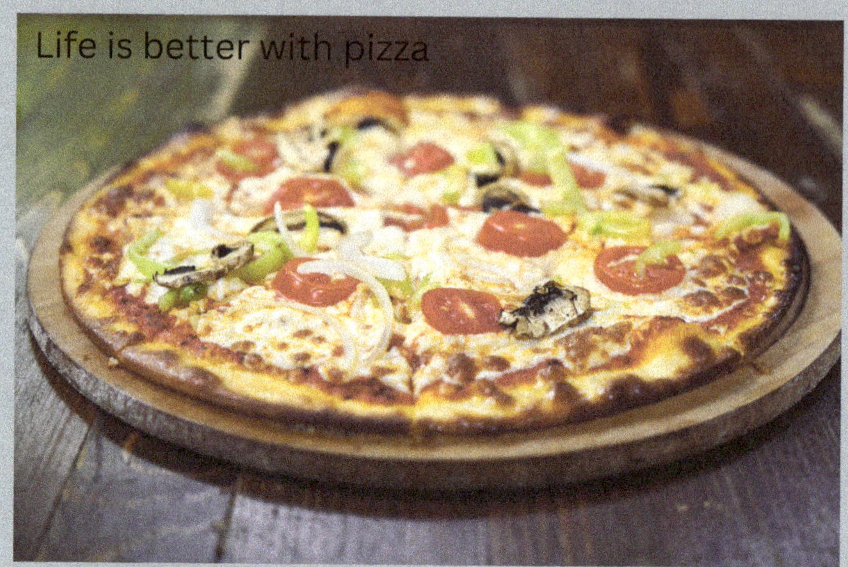

Let's face it, we've all been in the same predicament at one point. It's 2 a.m. and you should have gone to sleep 4 hours ago and now you just can't resist those deliciously tempting, but not-so-healthy foods. But don't worry, there's a way to indulge without feeling guilty (well, maybe just a little guilty). Here are some tips on how to eat the wrong foods the right way:

I Ooh La Pizza, the ultimate comfort food. The savory combination of bread, cheese, sauce, sausages, and, and, and… But instead of inhaling the entire pie in one sitting, try to savor each slice slowly. And if you're feeling really fancy, use a knife and fork to make it seem like a classy affair. Plus, you'll feel like you're dining at a fancy Italian restaurant, even if you're really just chlling on your couch in your sweatpants. Bonus points if you decide to pair it with a glass of wine.

II The crispy, salty golden goodness of French fries is the hardest to resist. But instead of dousing them in ketchup or ranch, try dipping them in a healthier sauce like hummus or guacamole. Not only will you get some extra nutrients, but you'll also feel fancy AF.

III Ice Cream is the ultimate cure for a bad day, but it's also a sneaky saboteur of your weight loss goals. Instead of eating it straight out of the tub, try scooping a reasonable amount into a bowl and topping it with fresh fruit and/or nuts. You'll still get the satisfaction of that sweet, creamy goodness with a healthy twist.

IV Chips and Dip are the perfect party snack, but they're also a recipe for a diet disaster if you are not portion conscious. Instead of mindlessly dipping, try putting a small amount of your chips and dip onto a plate. And if you're feeling extra bougie, use a fancy platter and fancy napkins to make it seem like a billionaire appetizer.

V Chocolate is the ultimate temptation, but it's also packed with antioxidants and can actually be good for you in moderation. So instead of scarfing down an entire chocolate bar because it's the one time a month when you want to eat the entire aisle, try savoring a small piece slowly. And if you want to feel real fancy, pair it with a glass of red wine, champagne or a cup of tea to give it that extra je ne sais quoi.

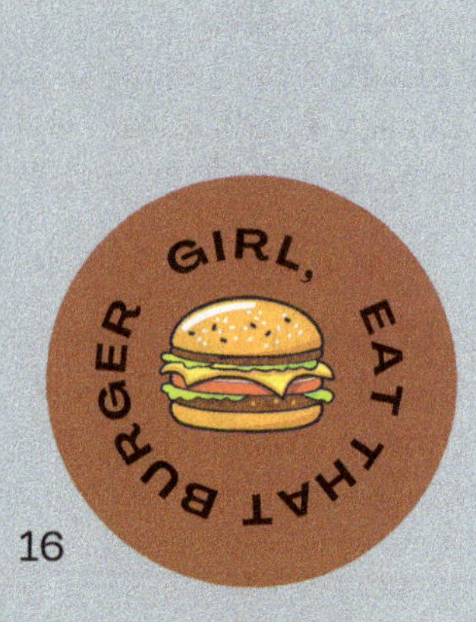

Chapter III

The Late-Night Fast: How to Avoid the Midnight Munchies

and Still Have Fun...Without Making Your Blood Pressure Skyrocket

Look, I get it. It's 10 pm and you're scrolling through Instagram, drooling over pictures of food, and suddenly the hunger monster strikes. Fear not for I have a solution that doesn't involve gnawing on your arm like a ravenous raccoon.

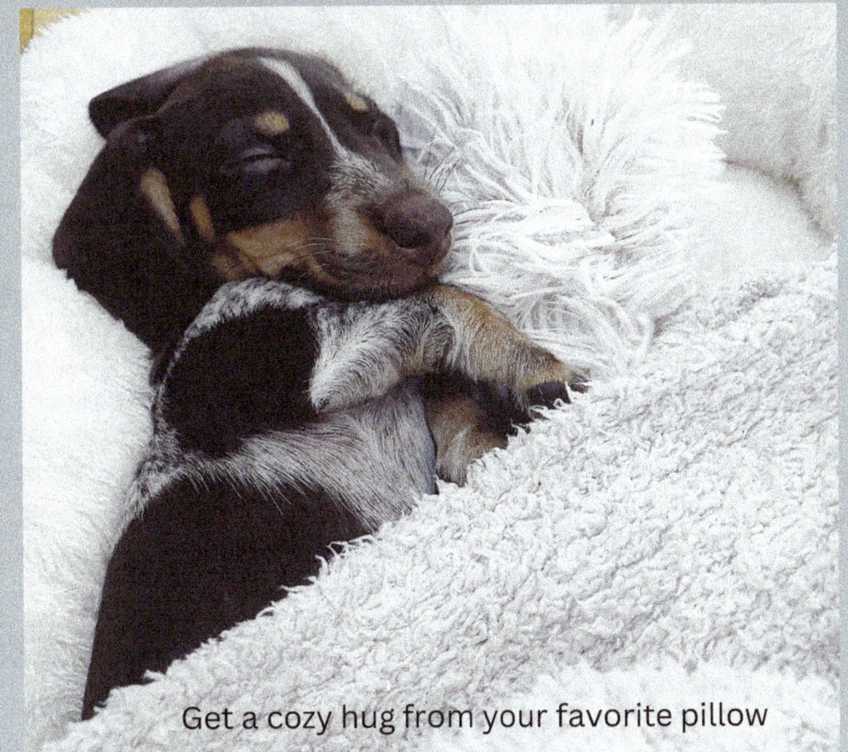

Get a cozy hug from your favorite pillow

The key to avoiding the midnight munchies is a little something I like to call the late-night fast. Here's how to do it without making your blood pressure shoot through the roof.

I Turn It into a Game. Make a bet with your friends or family on who can go the longest without eating after 8 pm. Why suffer in silence when you can turn your late-night fast into a fun challenge and make them suffer with you? Just make sure you bet something you're willing to lose unless you're confident in your willpower.

II Keep Your Mind Busy. When you're hungry, it's easy to think of nothing but food. Binge-watch a series, read a book, or write in a journal about your day & jot down new recipes you would like to try that you saw on TikTok. Or you can keep walking to the fridge trying to convince yourself not to grab a snack. At least you're getting steps in.

III Find Alternative Ways to Indulge Just because you're fasting doesn't mean you have to deprive yourself of all pleasure. Find alternative ways to indulge your senses, like taking a hot bubble bath, lighting some scented candles, listening to your favorite tunes, or just sitting in silence.

IV Don't Sacrifice Sleep for Snacks. If all else fails, just go to bed. You won't be able to eat if you're unconsciously drooling. Not to mention, you'll wake up feeling refreshed and ready to tackle the day and a meal. Just make sure you don't oversleep and miss your alarm, or you'll end up fasting until lunchtime.

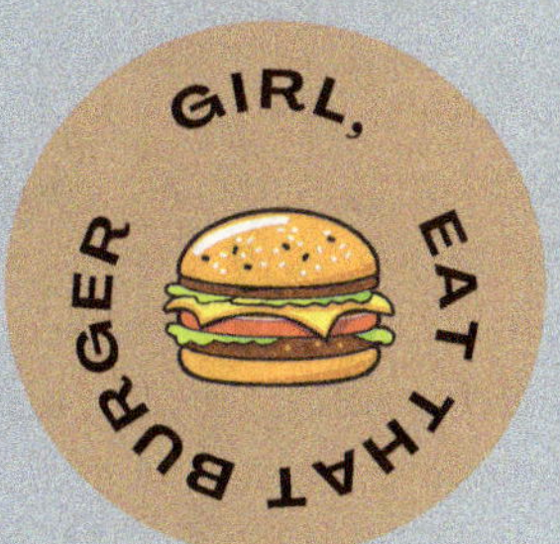

Chapter IV

Meal Planning: Because Life is Too Short for Bland Diets

The healthier alternative to fried chicken.

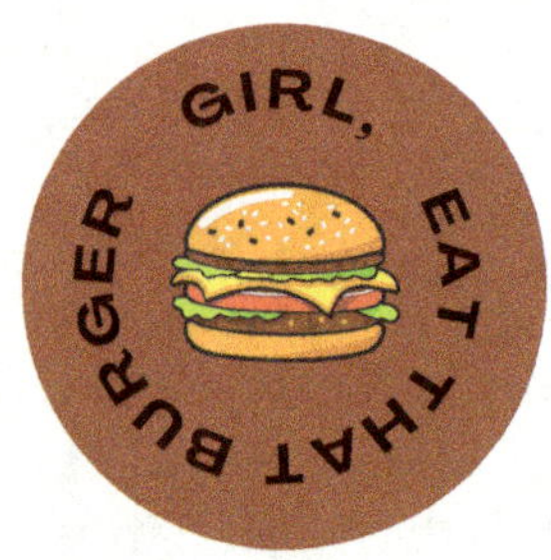

Meal planning is the key to success when it comes to losing weight. But let's be real, the thought of eating fish and salad every day for the rest of your life is about as appealing as watching paint dry.

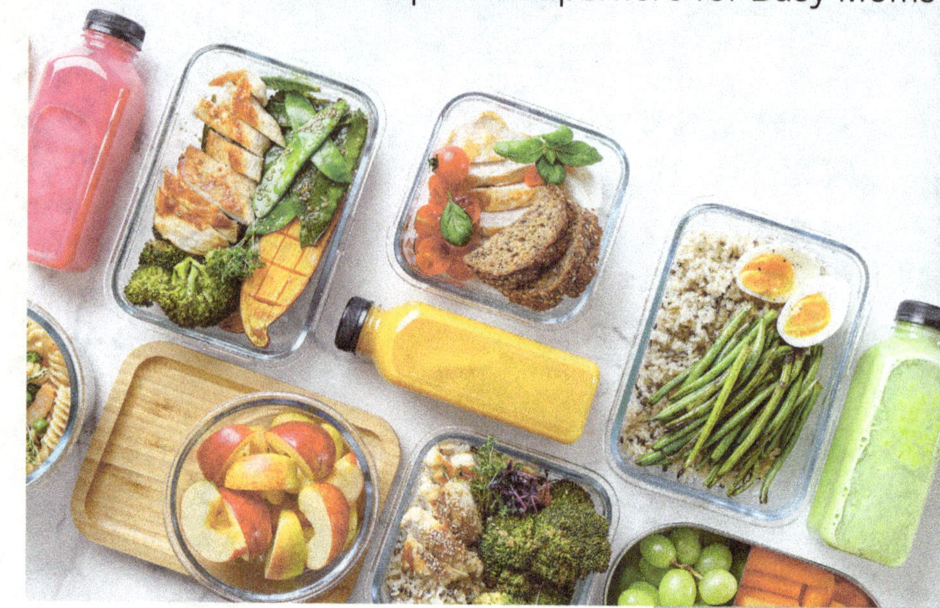

I Embrace Variety Say goodbye to boring salads and hello to a world of exciting flavors. Experiment with different cuisines, spices, and ingredients to keep your taste buds on their toes. One day you could be enjoying a spicy Thai curry, the next a flavorful Mediterranean dish. Who says losing weight has to be bland and boring?

II Don't Be Afraid to Cheat (a Little) We all have our guilty pleasures. Maybe it's a slice of pizza or a bowl of ice cream. The key is to indulge in moderation. Add a little treat to your meal plan once a week to keep things interesting and satisfying. Just don't go overboard and end up in a food coma.

III Get Creative with Meal Prep Meal prep doesn't have to mean slaving over a hot stove for hours on end. Get creative with your meal prep by making it fun. Turn on some music, dance around the kitchen, and get chopping. Plus, when you have healthy, delicious meals waiting for you in the fridge, you'll be less tempted to reach for the fast food menu.

IV Don't Overthink It Sometimes the best meals are the simplest. Don't stress out about making every meal a masterpiece. Just focus on making healthy, satisfying meals that you enjoy. And if you end up eating the same thing for lunch every day for a week, that's okay. Life is too short to stress about every little thing.

V Spice It Up No one wants to eat plain chicken and broccoli for every meal. It's like a party with no music – a total snooze-fest. Add some spice to your life (and your meals) with different herbs, spices, and seasonings. Your taste buds will thank you, and you'll avoid falling asleep at the dinner table.

Chapter V

How to Outsmart Your Cravings

Don't Give in to the Dark Side

Picture this: you're minding your own business, going about your day, and suddenly it hits you - a craving for something so deliciously sinful, it's like the devil himself is whispering in your ear saying eat something sweet, salty, or greasy. But fear not because with these sneaky strategies, you'll be able to outsmart your cravings.

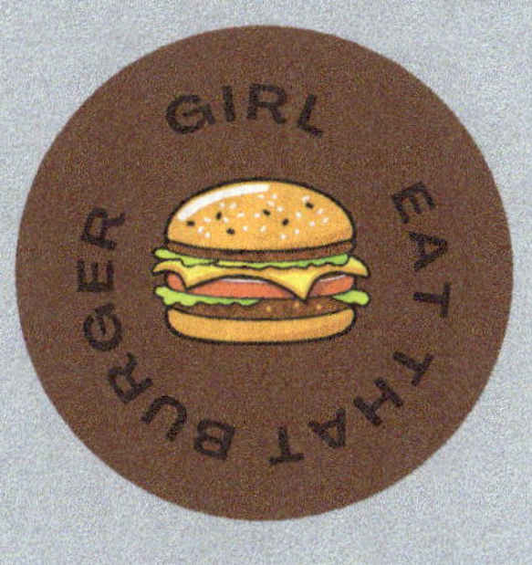

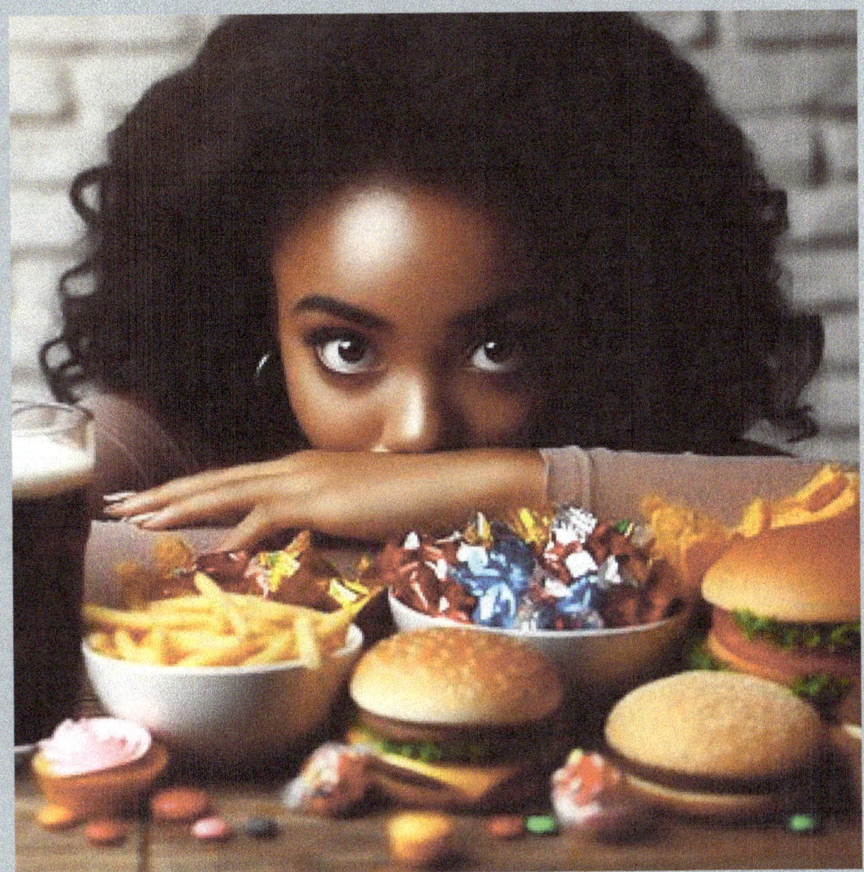

I Play Mind Games. Cravings are like the playground bully - they only have power if you let them. So, play some mind games and outsmart those pesky cravings. Visualize yourself triumphantly saying "no" to that slice of pizza, or call up a friend because those conversations can last for hours.. Trust me, it works.

II Have a Snack Attack. If you're feeling like a little snack, make sure you have some healthy snacks on hand to satisfy your cravings. Keep some nuts, fruits, or veggies within arm's reach to fend off those sneaky little cravings.

III Drink Your Problems Away! No, I'm not talking about alcohol (although a little glass of red wine never hurt anyone). I'm talking about water, baby. Drinking water can help you feel full and satisfied, which means fewer cravings. Plus, it's good for your health and your skin. Win-win.

IV Get a Little Spicy Add some spice to your meals, and you might just find that you're less likely to crave junk food. Spicy foods can increase your metabolism and make you feel fuller, so you're less likely to snack on junk food.

V Avoid the Triggers. If you're easily tempted, stay away from the things that trigger your cravings. Don't walk down the candy and chip aisle at the grocery store. Try to avoid the vending machine at work. It might be tough at first, but trust me, it's worth it and it works.

Chapter VI

The Lazy Person's Guide to Sweating

Sweat and have fun while doing it.

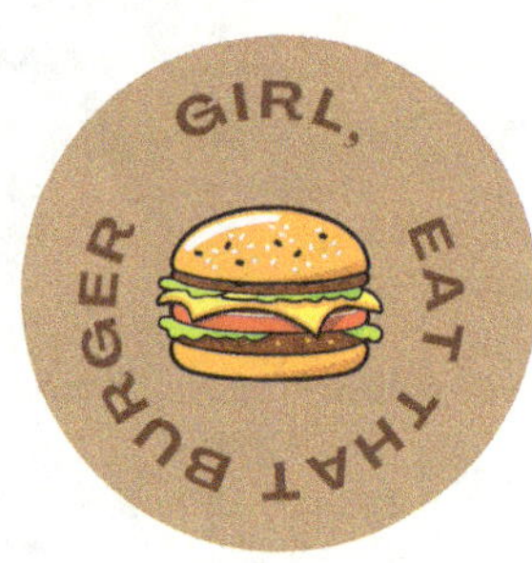

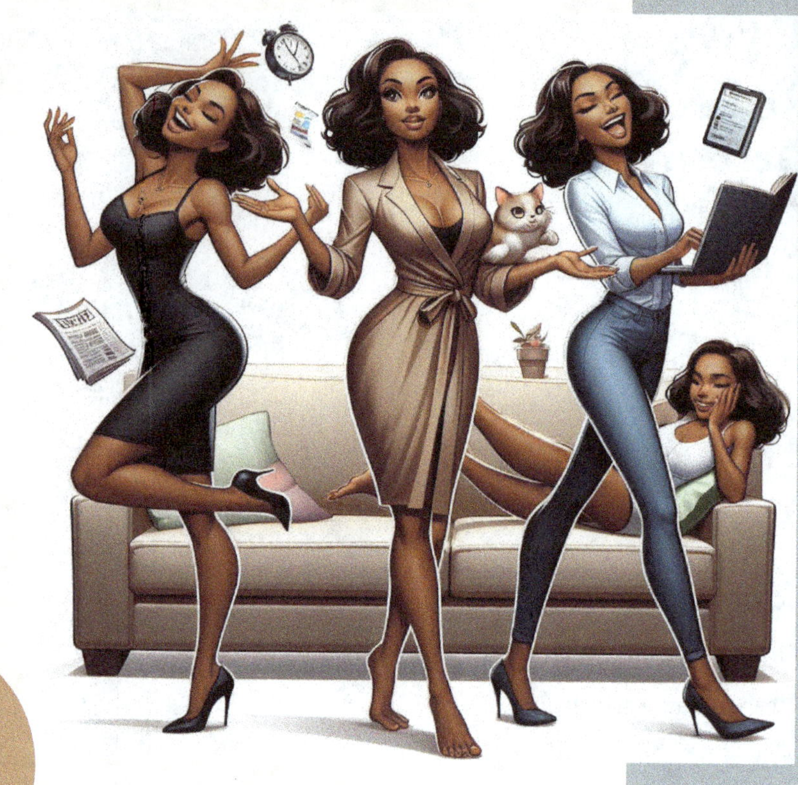

Let's be honest, exercising can be a real drag. But fear not, my fellow Ravishing Recliner Royal Regals, for I have compiled a list of non-exercises that will have you sweating without ever leaving your comfort zone.

I Laughing Your Butt Off (Literally) Have you ever had a laughing fit so hard that your stomach hurt? Well, turns out that laughing actually burns calories! So, grab some friends, watch a funny movie or stand-up comedy, and let the laughs roll. Bonus points if you can make it a full-on ab workout by doing some crunches while you giggle.

II Netflix and Sweat (With a Partner, If You're Lucky) Why hit the gym when you can get a full-body workout from the comfort of your own couch? Not only does it get your heart rate up, but it also works your muscles. Plus, let's be real, it's a lot more fun than doing squats. So, get your partner on board and turn up the heat (literally and figuratively).

III Dance Like a Fool (And Get Fit While You're at It) You don't have to be a professional dancer to bust a move and burn some calories. Whether you're doing the cha-cha slide or twerking like Miley Cyrus, you'll be burning calories and having fun. And who knows, maybe you'll even impress that cute guy or girl or hell, even yourself!

Chapter VII

Lifestyle Changes - From Couch Potato to Kale Crusader

Instead of satisfying your sweet tooth challenge yourself with a hassle-free treat.

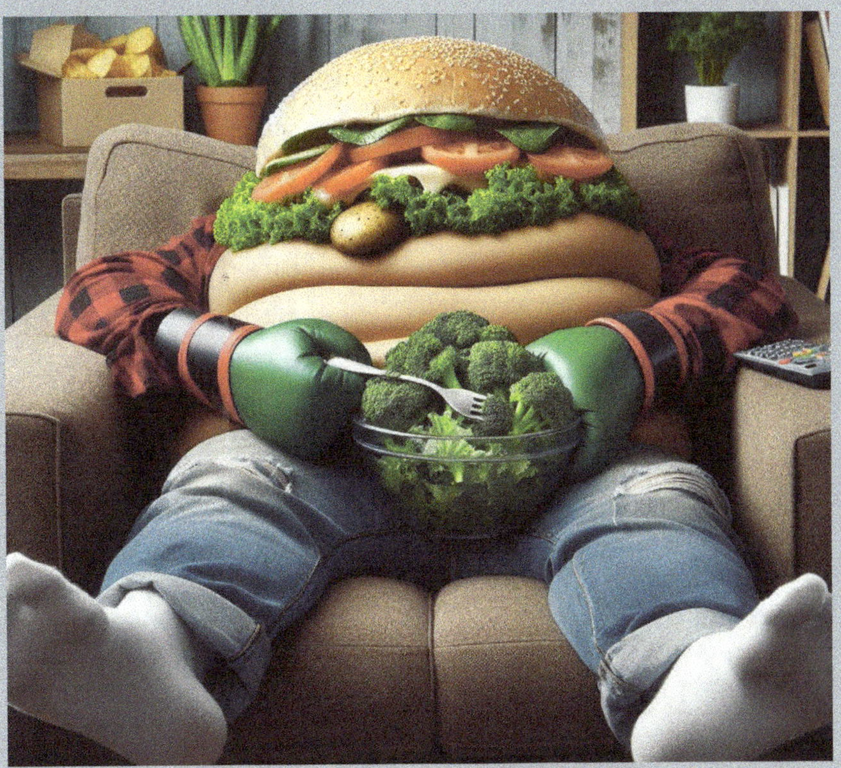

Let's face it, changing your lifestyle can be as appealing as eating a raw potato. But if you want to keep that weight off, you gotta do what you gotta do. So, let's get started with some hilarious tips and tricks to make the transition as smooth as possible.

I Find Exercise You Actually Enjoy (Yes, It Exists!) First things first, let's talk about exercise. I know, I know - it's not always the most exciting thing in the world, right? But the key is to find something you actually enjoy. Hate running? Try dancing! Can't stand the gym? Go for a hike! The options are endless.

II Treat Yo' Self , don't cheat Yo' Self. I get it, sometimes you just need a good ol' fashioned treat. Don't restrict yourself, but you gotta do it in moderation girl. So, go ahead and indulge in that slice of pizza or that piece of cake. But remember, one slice does not equal the whole damn cake. Moderation is key!

III Recruit Your Squad! Changing your lifestyle is tough, but it's a whole lot easier when you have some support. Recruit your friends and family to join you on this journey. Not only will it make things more fun, but it'll also keep you accountable. Plus, there's nothing like a little friendly competition to spice things up.

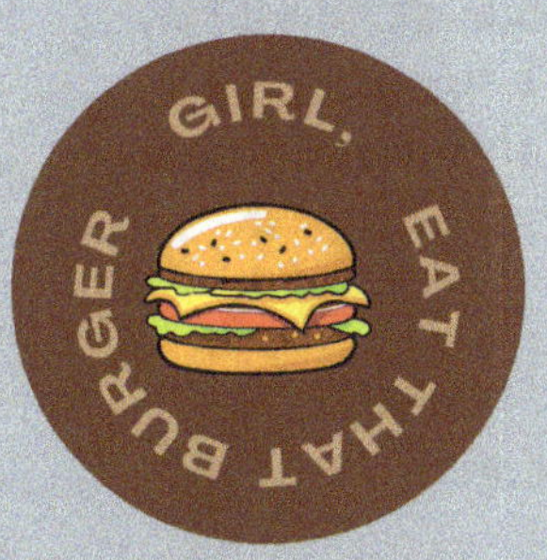

Chapter VIII

Water, Sleep, and Stress - Oh My!

The fun killers.

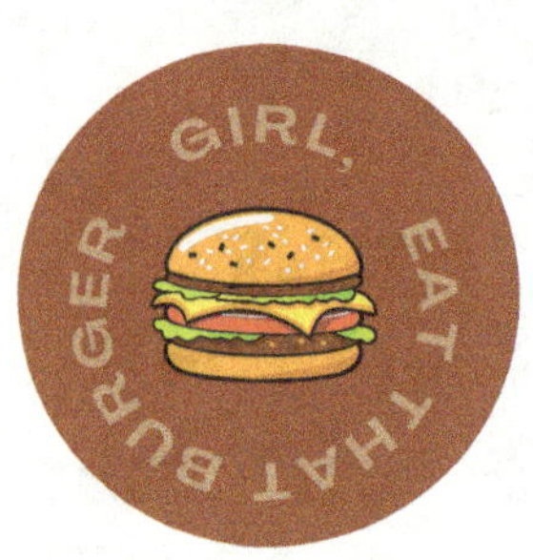

When it comes to weight loss, staying hydrated is crucial. But it's not just about drinking your daily dose of H2O - it's about managing your sleep and stress levels too. So, let's dive into why water, sleep, and stress management are so important, and how you can make sure you're keeping yourself properly hydrated, rested, and relaxed.

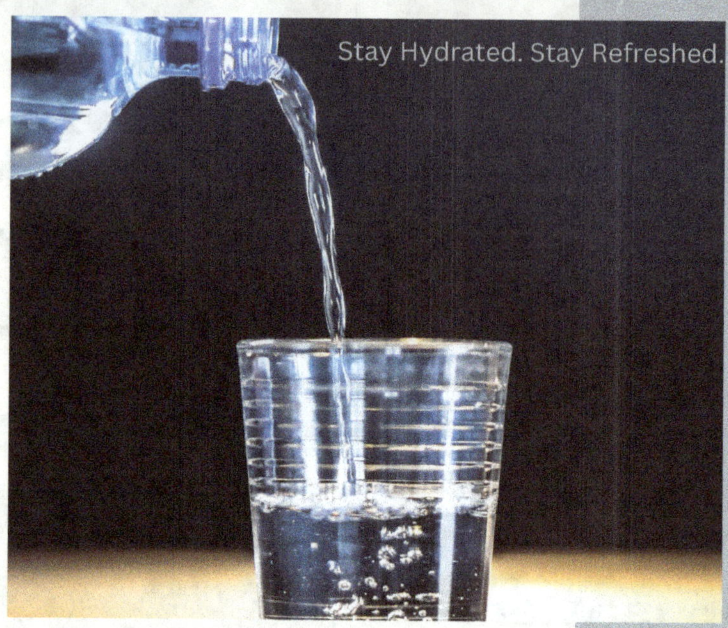

I Water, Water, Water Let's all get wasted. (And You Should Be Drinking It All) First things first, let's talk about the importance of water. Not only does it keep you hydrated, but it can also help you feel fuller, boost your metabolism, and flush out toxins. Plus, if you're like me and love to snack, drinking water can help curb those pesky little attacks.

II Guess what girl? Did you know that drinking water is only effective if you're actually drinking it? So, make sure you're staying hydrated throughout the day. Keep a water bottle with you at all times and take sips regularly. Don't forget to mix things up - try infusing your water with fruit for a little added pizazz.

III Snooze Your Way to Success (Literally) Now, let's talk about sleep. Getting enough shut-eye is crucial for weight loss. When you're sleep-deprived, your body produces more of the hormone ghrelin (which makes you feel hungry) and less of the hormone leptin (which makes you feel full). Plus, when you're tired, you're more likely to reach for high-calorie snacks for a quick energy boost. So, make sure you're getting those Zzzs. Get that beauty sleep. Aim for seven to eight hours of sleep every night and establish a bedtime routine to help you wind down. Avoid caffeine and electronics before bed. Try reading a book or taking a warm bath instead.

IV Stress Less, Weigh Less (Seriously) and most importantly, let's talk about stress. When you're stressed, your body releases the hormone cortisol, which can lead to increased hunger and cravings for high-calorie foods. So, if you want to lose weight, you need to manage your stress levels. Remember the Serenity Prayers during these difficult times.

V Find activities that help you unwind, like yoga, meditation, or listening to music. And if all else fails, just sex it off. Studies show that sex can reduce stress levels, boost your mood and from what I've heard, most people are happy afterwards, Wink Wink.

Chapter IX

Concluded Conclusions

**Faith is not about jumping to conclusions, it's about concluding to jump.
W. T. Purkiser**

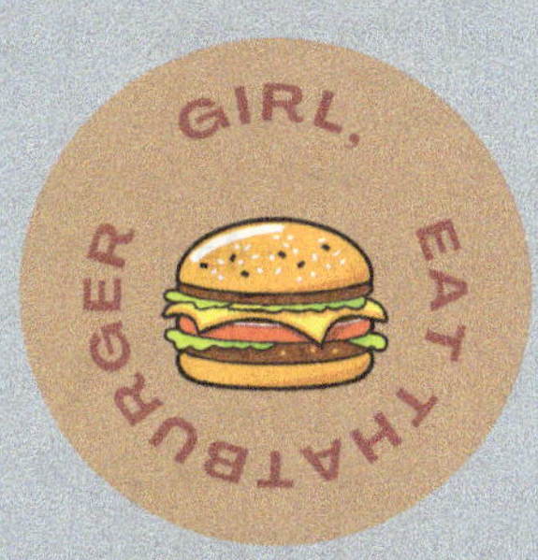

Ok Ladies, there you have it. A comprehensive guide to losing weight by changing simple things to improve your lifestyle. We covered everything from laughing your way to a six-pack to parking far away when you know you're about to misbehave. Remember to take baby steps and try one thing at a time if changing several things will give you anxiety.

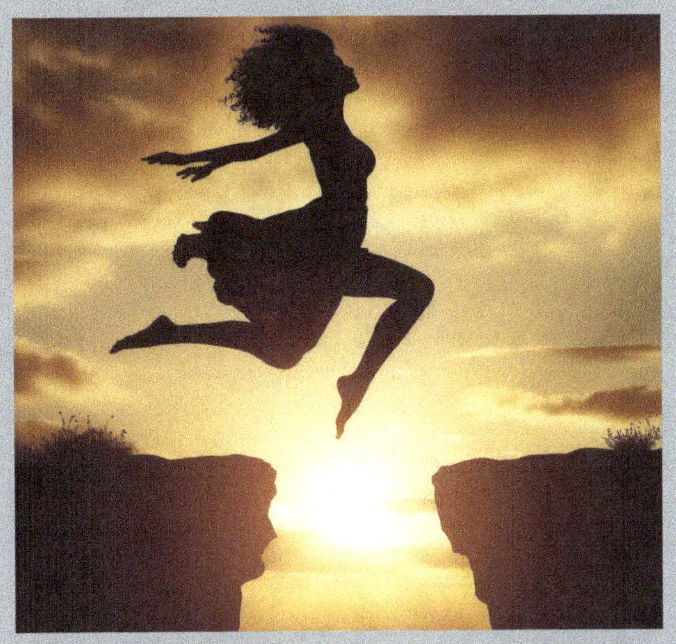

I Now ladies, let me remind you that despite us being in this together, I am not a licensed dietician or personal trainer. So, please do consult with your doctor before you start any new weight loss program. Because, let's be honest, you wouldn't want to end up with buns of steel and high blood pressure. After all, everyone's body is different, and what works for me might not work for you.

II This weight loss journey is not a marathon it's a destination. You might slip up and eat a whole cake once in a while, but that's okay! Just remember to dust off the crumbs, get back on track, and keep laughing along the way. Because laughter burns calories, and a good sense of humor is the secret sauce to a healthy lifestyle. Keep in mind that you are human and entitled to make mistakes.

III In the end, the key to losing weight is finding what works best for you and your lifestyle. Noone else. So, whether you're a gym rat or a couch potato, there's a way for you to shed those unwanted pounds and embrace a healthier lifestyle. And remember, it's not about being perfect or depriving yourself of the things you love. It's about making small, sustainable changes that add up over time.

IV So go forth, my fellow big back warriors, and embrace the power of laughter, love, and a few extra steps to the grocery store. And remember, if all else fails, just wear black and blame it on the lighting. Cheers to a healthier, funnier you! Don't forget to laugh, sweat and hydrate along the way.

Chapter X

KEY TAKEAWAYS

Let's revisit some things to remember from each chapter.

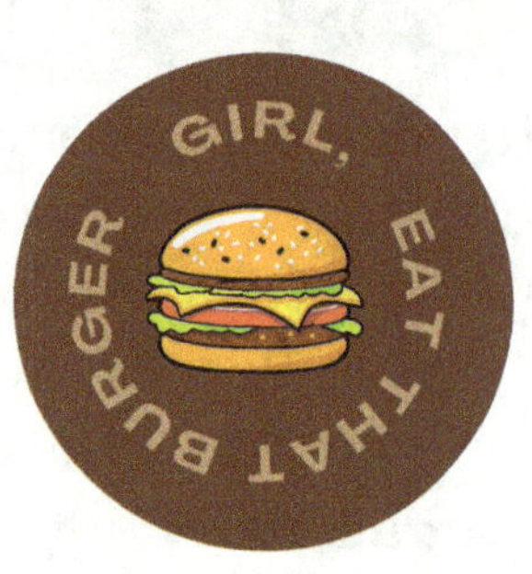

Remember it only takes 30 days to form new habits. Good habits are positive behaviors that we consistently practice. They contribute to our overall well-being and help us achieve our goals.

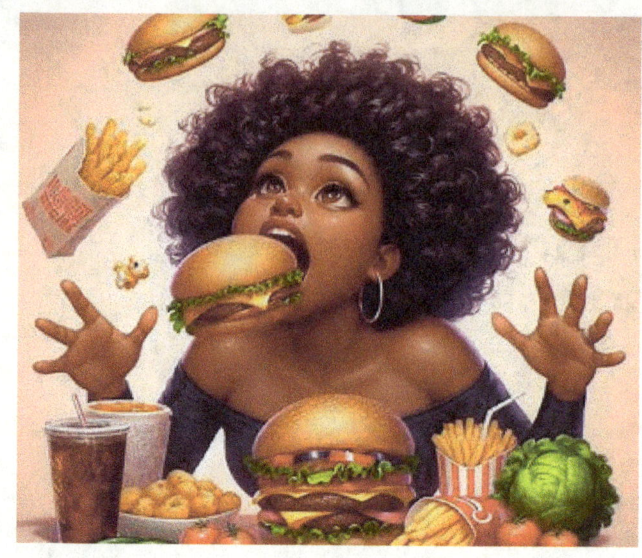

I Next time you find yourself mindlessly eating, take a step back and remember these sneaky culprits and ask yourself why. Are you hungry, or are you just bored or could it be stress? By identifying and addressing the root causes of your overeating, you'll be one step closer to achieving your weight loss goals. And remember, if all else fails, there's always celery sticks. But who the heck like those?

II Eating the wrong foods doesn't have to be a guilt trip. By making conscious choices and indulging in moderation, you can enjoy your favorite foods without sacrificing your health goals. And while you're at it pretend its gourmet and maybe you'll even feel a little fancy while indulging.

III The late-night fast doesn't have to be a painful experience. With a little creativity, distraction, and self-discipline, you can avoid the midnight munchies and still have fun. Just don't forget to consult with your doctor before starting any fasting routine.

IV Remember, meal planning is all about finding a balance between healthy eating and enjoying life. So, don't be afraid to get creative and experiment with new flavors, ingredients and recipes. Consult with your doctor or nutritionist before starting any new meal plan or diet. They may even have some delicious recipe recommendations of their own!

V By using these sneaky little strategies, you'll be able to outsmart your cravings. Don't forget, it's okay to indulge every once in a while. Just make sure you don't end up in a sugar coma. Now, go forth and rebel against those cravings! Find healthy alternatives, sometimes, all we need is a little crunch or sweetness to satisfy a craving. Instead of reaching for chips or candy, try snacking on some baby carrots, sliced apples, or air-popped popcorn. Your taste buds and waistline will thank you.

MORE
TAKEAWAYS

**More things to
remember**

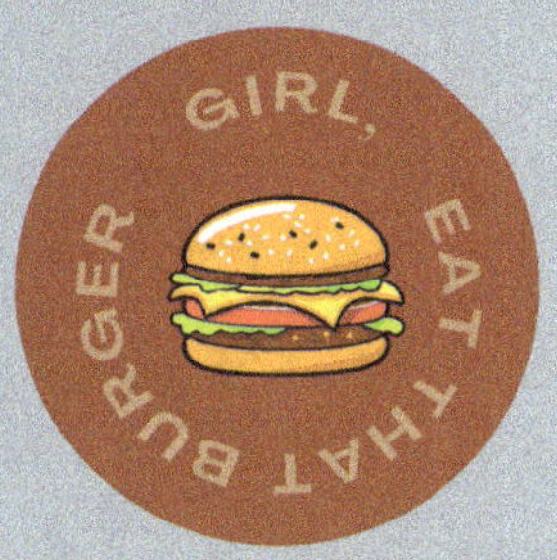

"Just believe in yourself.
Even if you don't, pretend
that you do and, at some
point, you will."
– Venus Williams

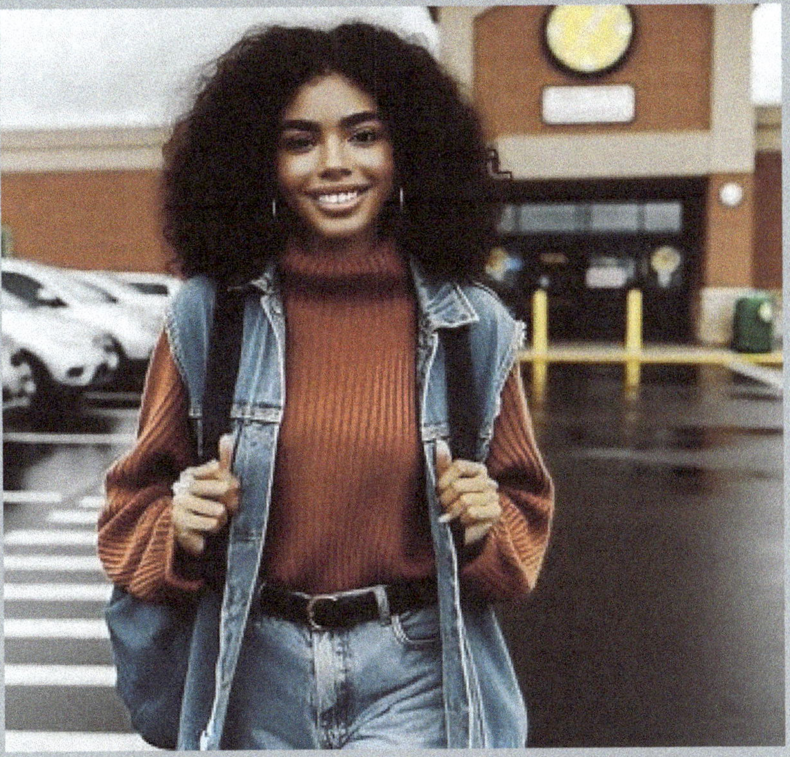

VI Laugh Your Way to a Six-Pack Who needs crunches when you can just laugh your way to a toned tummy? It's simple, really. Just queue up your favorite comedy special, grab some popcorn (air-popped, of course), and prepare to giggle your way to six-pack city.

VII Take the Stairs (And Pretend You're Climbing Mount Everest) Why waste your time on the stair-stepper when you can get a workout just by taking the stairs? And to make it even more exciting, pretend you're scaling Mount Everest as you ascend each step. Don't forget to bring a water bottle and some oxygen, just in case.

VIII Park Far Away (And Walk Like You Mean It) Who needs a parking spot close to the entrance when you can burn some calories by parking at the other end of the lot? And to make it even more challenging, walk like you're running late to catch the last train out of town. You'll be sweating in no time

IX For example, if you're craving a burger, opt for a lettuce wrap instead of a bun. Want something sweet? Have a piece of fruit instead of a candy bar. And if you do want to indulge every once in a while, go for it! Just make sure to balance it out with healthy choices the rest of the time

X So, there you have it - the importance of water, sleep, and stress management during weight loss. Remember to drink your water, get your beauty sleep, and stress less. And if all else fails, just remember that a little laughter can go a long way.

In the end, the key to losing weight is finding what works best for you and your lifestyle. So, whether you're a gym rat or a couch potato, there's a way for you to shed those unwanted pounds and embrace a healthier lifestyle. And remember, it's not about being perfect or depriving yourself of the things you love. It's about making small, sustainable changes that add up over time.

31 Days of Quick High Metabolism Recipes to Unbig Your Back

99 RECIPES!

INCLUDED

BURGERS FOR DAYS

D.K.R.G.

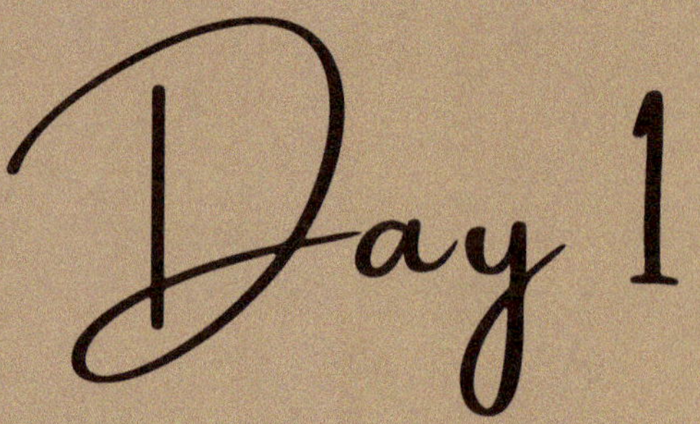

Day 1

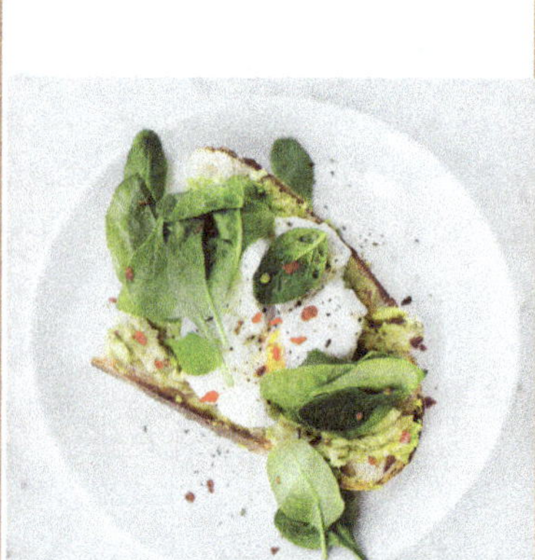

Avocado Toast
Ingredients:

- 2 slices whole grain bread
- 1 ripe avocado
- Salt, pepper, and red pepper flakes to taste
- Instructions: Mash the avocado and spread it on toasted bread. Season with salt, pepper, and red pepper flakes.

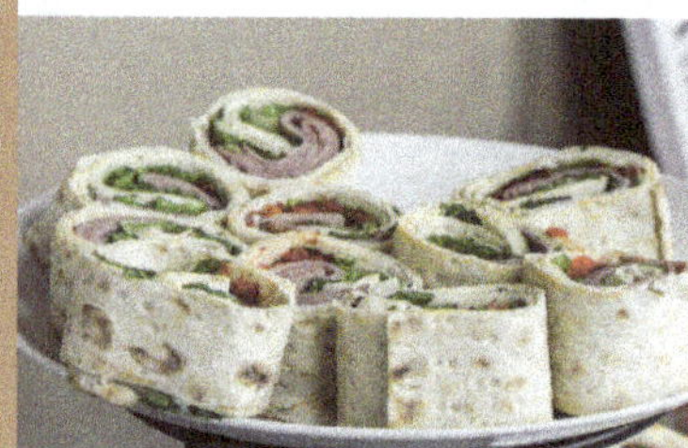

Turkey and Veggie Wrap
Ingredients:

- 1 whole wheat tortilla
- 3 oz. sliced turkey breast
- Mixed greens
- Sliced cucumber, tomato, and bell
- pepper
- Hummus
- Instructions: Layer the turkey, mixed greens, and sliced vegetables on the tortilla. Spread hummus, wrap tightly, and cut in half.

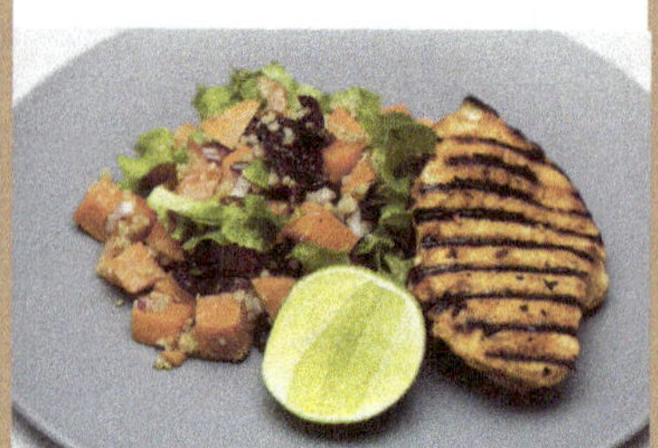

Grilled Lemon Herb Chicken with Quinoa
Ingredients:

- 4 oz. chicken breast
- Juice of 1 lemon
- 1 tsp olive oil

- Mixed herbs (rosemary, thyme, oregano)
- 1/2 cup cooked quinoa
- Instructions: Marinate chicken in lemon juice, olive oil, and herbs. Grill until cooked through. Serve with cooked quinoa.

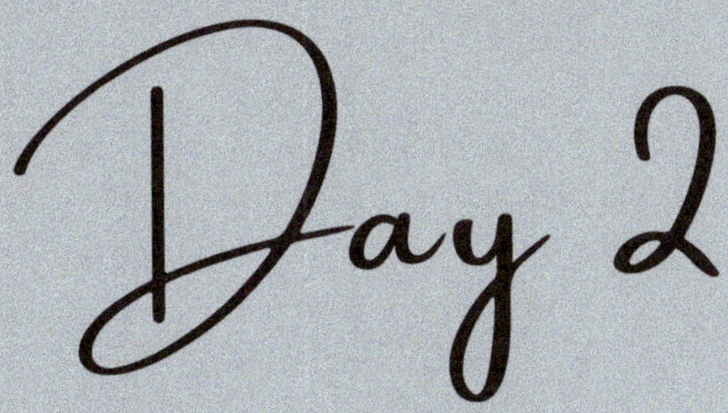

Day 2

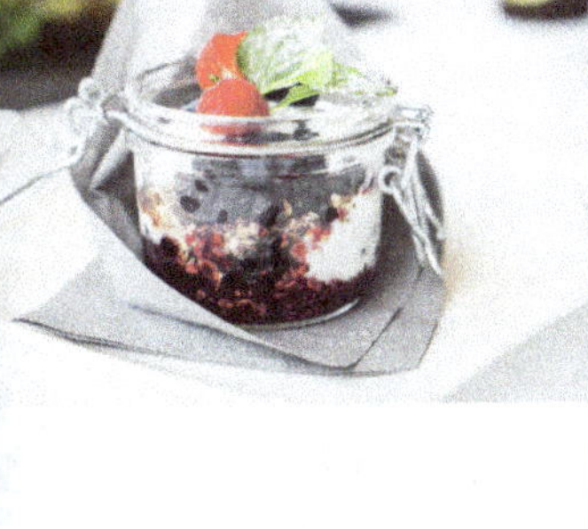

Greek Yogurt Parfait
Ingredients:
- 1 cup Greek yogurt
- 1/2 cup mixed berries
- 1/4 cup granola
- Instructions: Layer Greek yogurt, mixed berries, and granola in a glass or bowl.

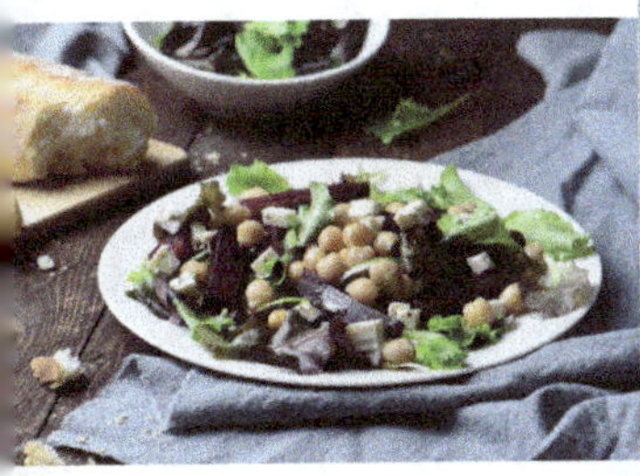

Chickpea Salad
Ingredients:
- 1 can chickpeas, drained and rinsed
- Diced cucumber, tomato, and red onion
- Chopped parsley
- Lemon juice and olive oil dressing
- Instructions: Combine all ingredients in a bowl and toss with dressing.

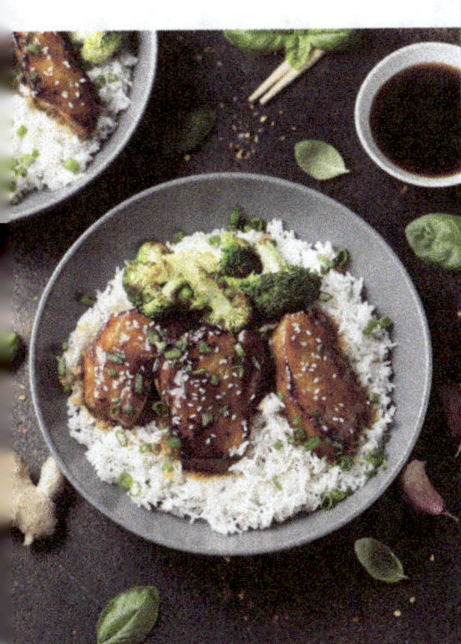

Teriyaki Salmon with Steamed Broccoli and Brown Rice
Ingredients:
- 4 oz. salmon fillet
- Teriyaki sauce
- 1 cup steamed broccoli
- 1/2 cup cooked brown rice
- Instructions: Marinate salmon in teriyaki sauce and bake until cooked through. Serve with steamed broccoli and brown rice.

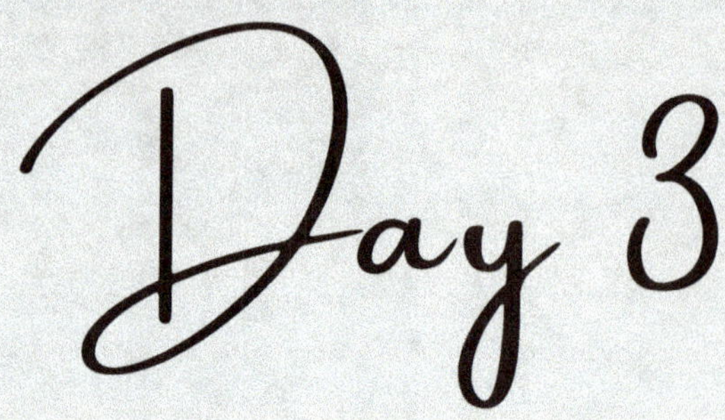

Day 3

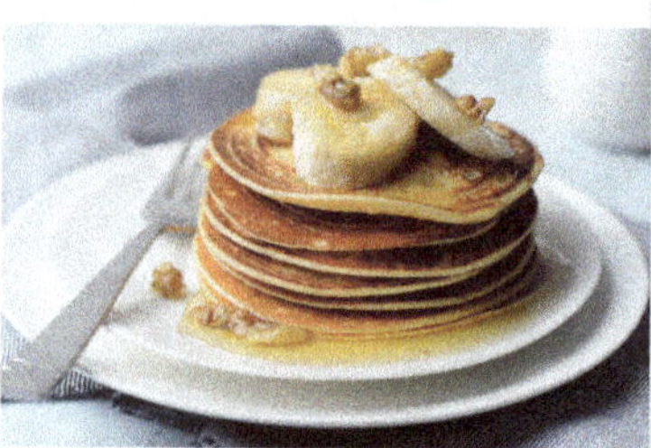

Banana Oat Pancakes
Ingredients:

- 1 ripe banana
- 1/2 cup rolled oats
- 1 egg
- Dash of cinnamon
- Instructions: Mash banana and mix with oats, egg, and cinnamon. Cook like regular pancakes.

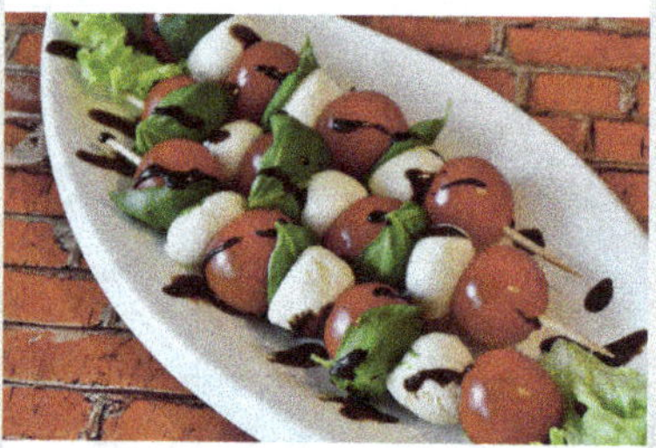

Caprese Salad
Ingredients:

- Sliced tomatoes
- Fresh mozzarella cheese
- Fresh basil leaves
- Balsamic glaze
- Instructions: Arrange sliced tomatoes, mozzarella, and basil on a plate. Drizzle with balsamic glaze.

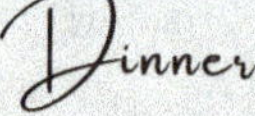
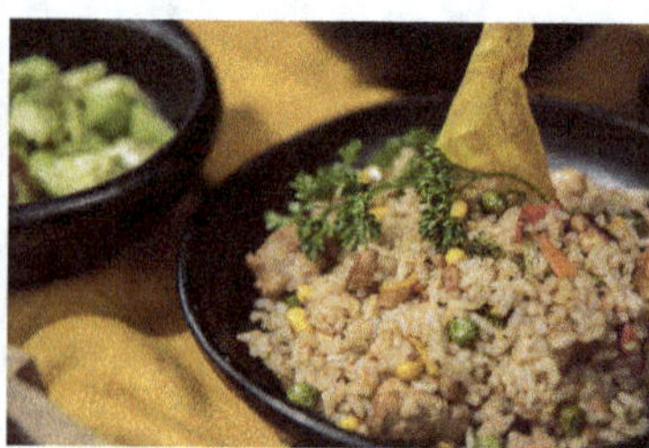

Stir-Fried Tofu with Vegetables and Cauliflower Rice
Ingredients:

- 4 oz. firm tofu, cubed
- Mixed vegetables (bell peppers, snap peas, carrots)
- Low-sodium soy sauce
- 1 cup cauliflower rice
- Instructions: Stir-fry tofu and vegetables in soy sauce. Serve over cauliflower rice.

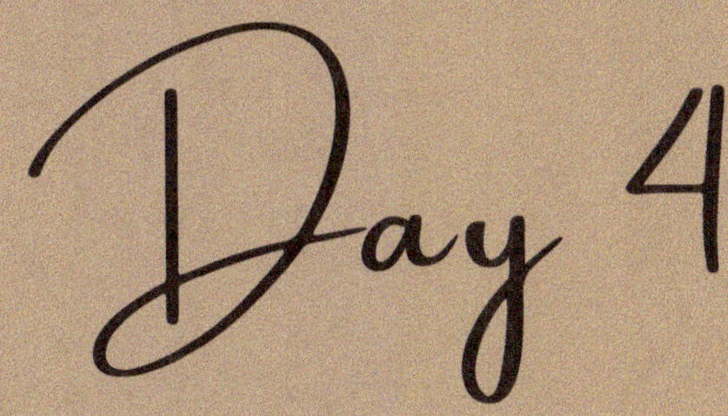

Day 4

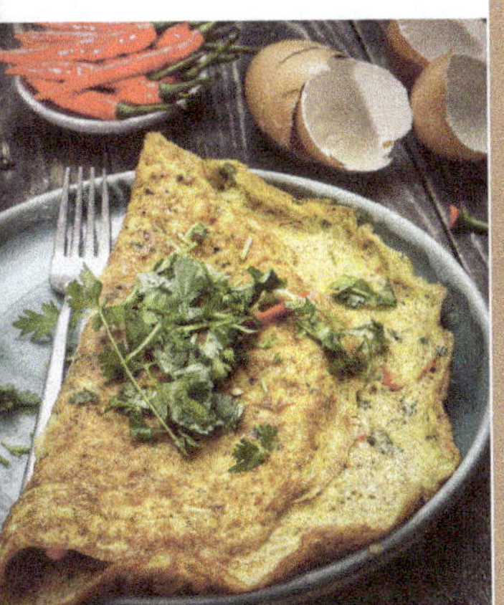

Veggie Omelette
Ingredients:
- 2 eggs
- Chopped bell peppers, onions, spinach
- Shredded cheese (optional)
- Instructions: Whisk eggs and pour into a hot skillet. Add vegetables and cheese, fold in half, and cook until set.

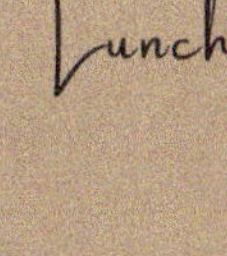

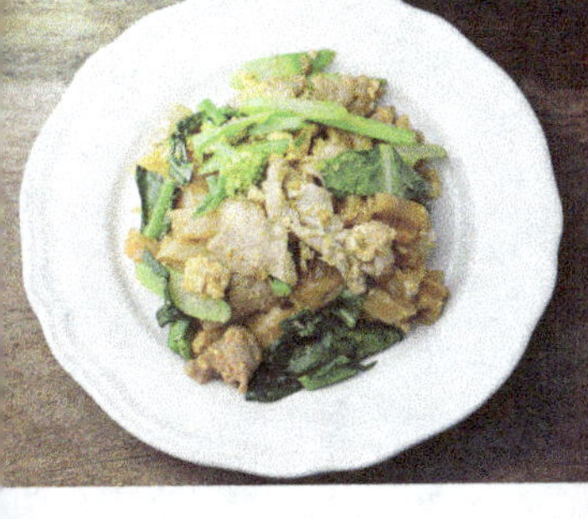

Turkey and Veggie Stir-Fry
Ingredients:
- Turkey breast strips
- Mixed vegetables (such as bell peppers, broccoli, carrots)
- Soy sauce
- Garlic, ginger, olive oil
- Instructions: Stir-fry turkey breast strips and mixed vegetables in olive oil with minced garlic and ginger. Add soy sauce and cook until turkey is cooked through and vegetables are tender.

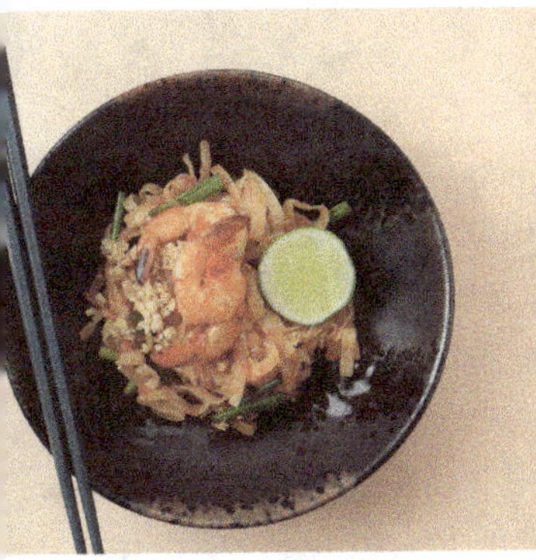

Shrimp Stir-Fry with Brown Rice Noodles
Ingredients:
- 4 oz. shrimp, peeled and deveined
- Stir-fry vegetables (broccoli, bell peppers, snap peas)
- Low-sodium stir-fry sauce
- 1 cup cooked brown rice noodles
- Instructions: Stir-fry shrimp and vegetables in sauce. Serve over cooked brown rice noodles.

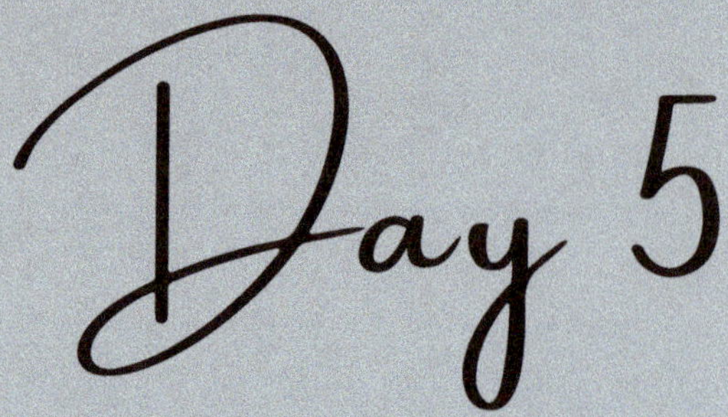

Breakfast

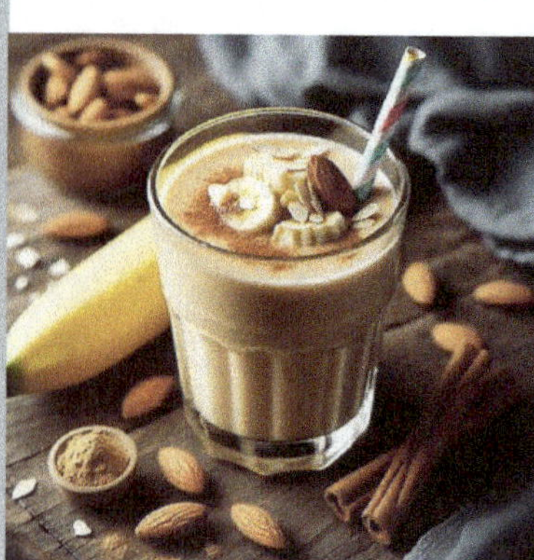

Peanut Butter Banana Smoothie
Ingredients:
- 1 ripe banana
- 1 tbsp peanut butter
- 1 cup almond milk
- Handful of spinach (optional)
- Instructions: Blend all ingredients until smooth.

Lunch

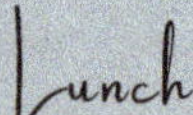

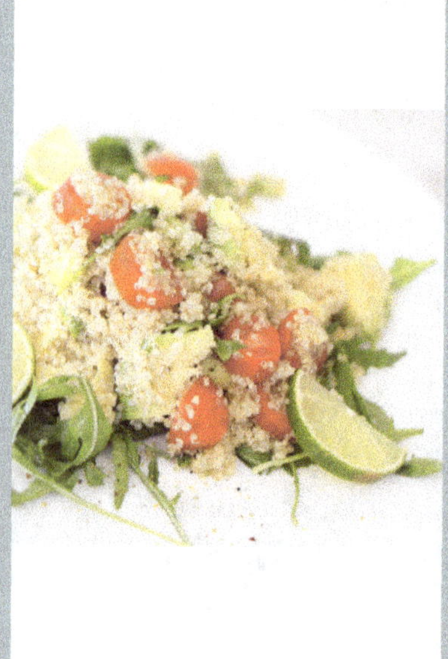

Quinoa Salad with Feta and Cherry Tomatoes
Ingredients:
- Cooked quinoa
- Cherry tomatoes, halved
- Crumbled feta cheese
- Chopped fresh parsley
- Lemon vinaigrette dressing
- Instructions: Combine all ingredients in a bowl and toss with dressing.

Dinner

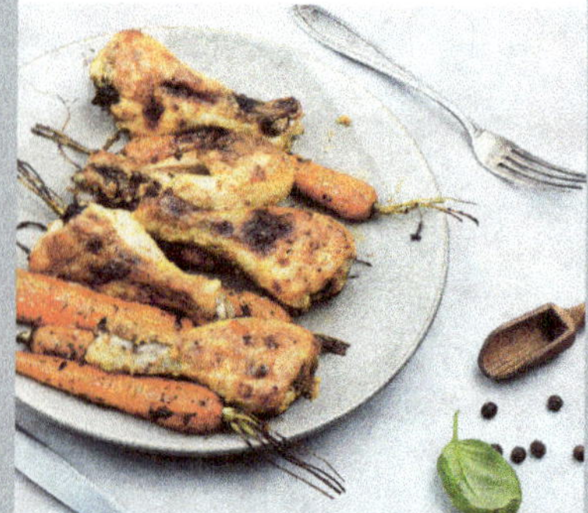

Baked Chicken Thighs with Roasted Vegetables
Ingredients:
- Chicken thighs
- Mixed vegetables (zucchini, bell peppers, onions)
- Olive oil
- Seasonings (garlic powder, paprika, Italian herbs)
- Instructions: Season chicken thighs and vegetables with olive oil and seasonings. Bake until chicken is cooked through and vegetables are tender.

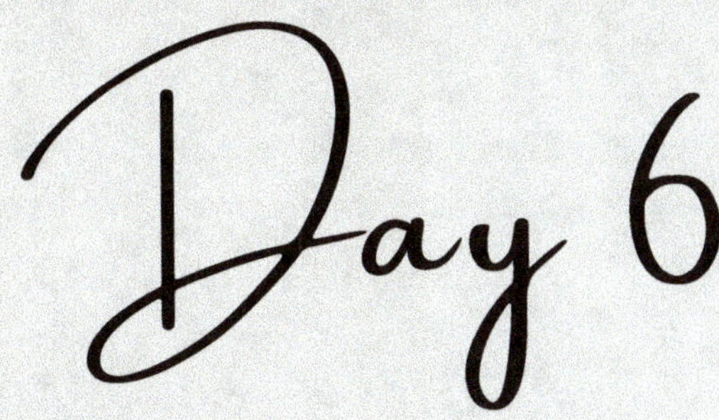

Day 6

Breakfast

Spinach and Mushroom Scramble
Ingredients:

- 2 eggs
- Handful of spinach
- Sliced mushrooms
- Shredded cheese (optional)
- Instructions: Scramble eggs in a skillet with spinach, mushrooms, and cheese until cooked through.

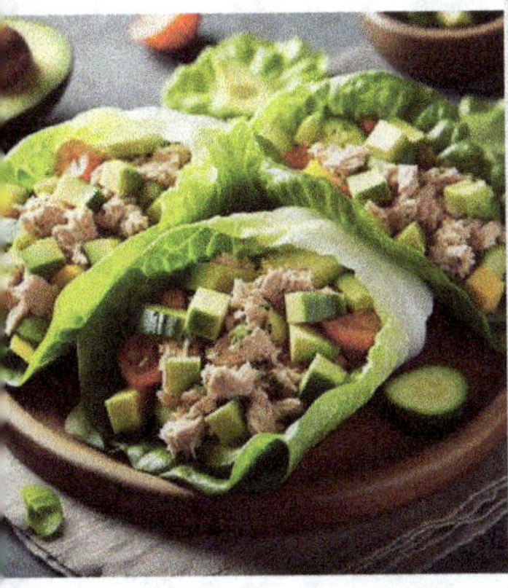

Lunch

Tuna Salad Lettuce Wraps
Ingredients:

- Canned tuna, drained
- Diced celery and red onion
- Greek yogurt or mayo
- Lettuce leaves
- Instructions: Mix tuna, celery, onion, and Greek yogurt or mayo. Spoon onto lettuce leaves and roll up.

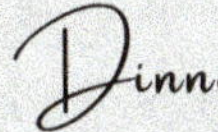

Dinner

Beef and Vegetable Stir-Fry with Cauliflower Rice
Ingredients:

- Lean beef strips
- Stir-fry vegetables (bell peppers,
- broccoli, carrots)
- Low-sodium stir-fry sauce
- 1 cup cauliflower rice
- Instructions: Stir-fry beef and vegetables in sauce. Serve over cooked cauliflower rice.

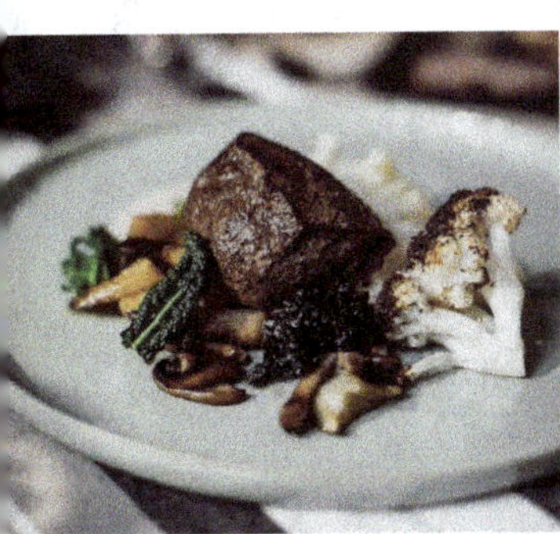

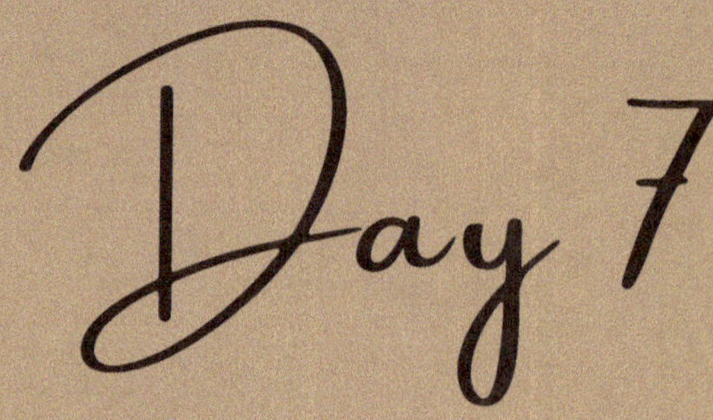

Day 7

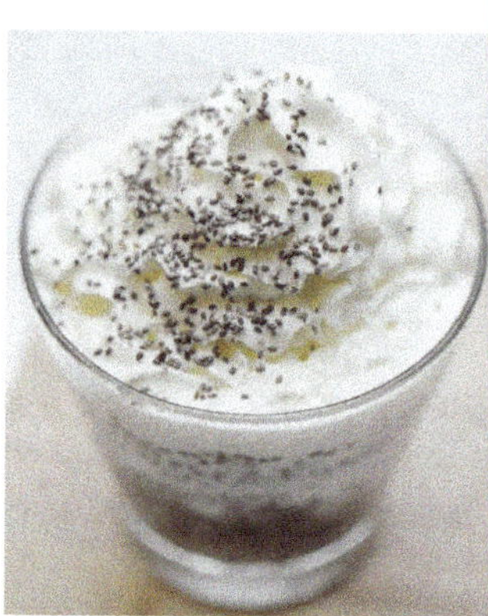

Breakfast

Chia Seed Pudding
Ingredients:
- 1/4 cup chia seeds
- 1 cup almond milk
- Vanilla extract
- Sweetener (honey, maple syrup)
- Instructions: Mix chia seeds, almond milk, vanilla, and sweetener. Let sit in the fridge overnight to thicken.

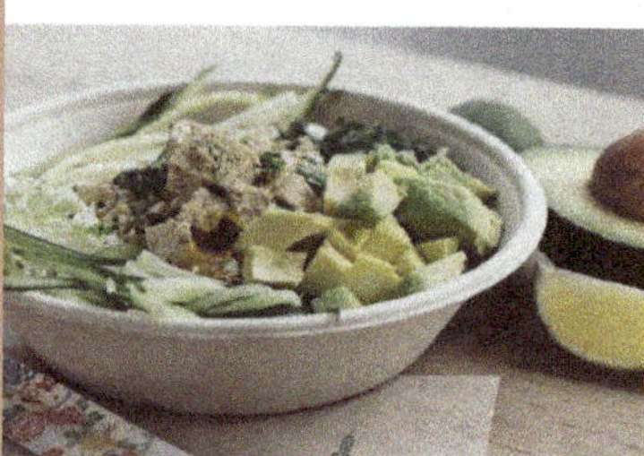

Lunch

Chicken and Avocado Salad
Ingredients:
- Grilled chicken breast, sliced
- Mixed greens
- Sliced avocado
- Cherry tomatoes
- Balsamic vinaigrette dressing
- Instructions: Toss all ingredients in a bowl with dressing.

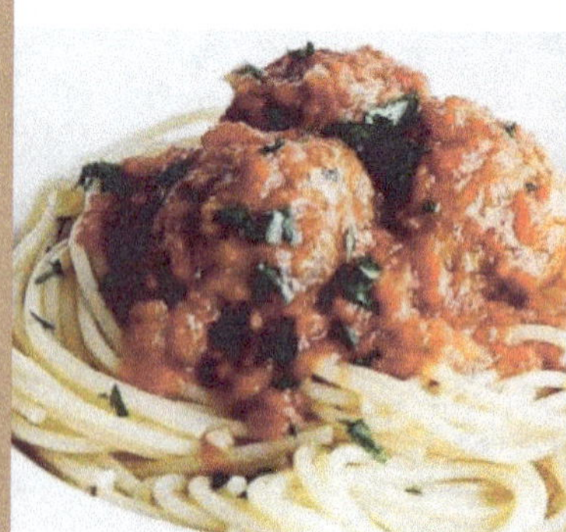

Dinner

Spaghetti Squash with Marinara Sauce and Turkey Meatballs
Ingredients:
- Roasted spaghetti squash
- Homemade or store-bought marinara
- sauce
- Turkey meatballs
- Instructions: Serve spaghetti squash topped with marinara sauce and turkey meatballs.

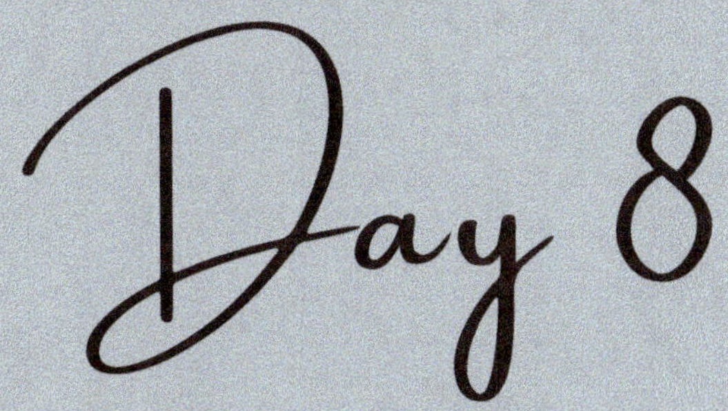

Day 8

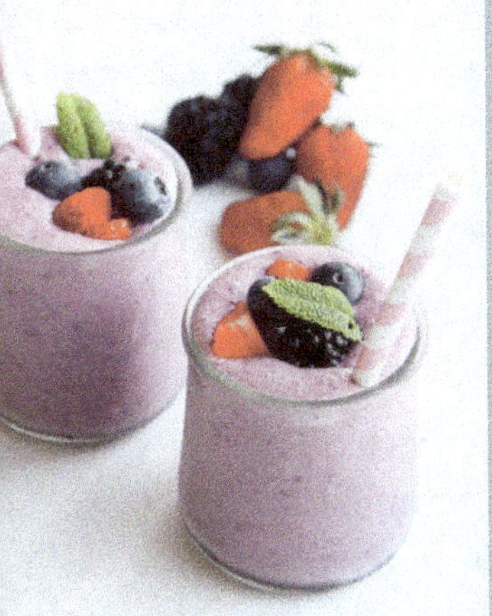

Berry Protein Smoothie Bowl
Ingredients:
- 1/2 cup frozen mixed berries
- 1/2 ripe banana
- 1/2 cup Greek yogurt
- 1 scoop protein powder (optional)
- Toppings: sliced strawberries, granola, chia seeds
- Instructions: Blend frozen berries, banana, Greek yogurt, and protein powder until smooth. Pour into a bowl and top with sliced strawberries, granola, and chia seeds.

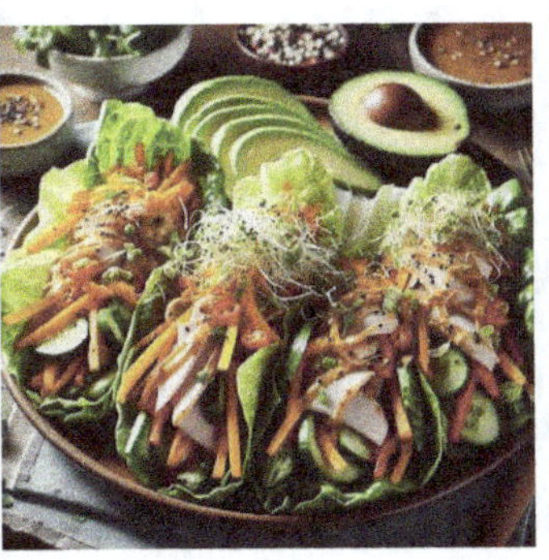

Turkey and Veggie Lettuce Wraps
Ingredients:
- Romaine lettuce leaves
- Sliced turkey breast
- Sliced cucumber, bell pepper, and avocado
- Dijon mustard or hummus
- Instructions: Spread mustard or hummus on lettuce leaves. Layer with turkey slices, sliced vegetables, and avocado. Roll up and enjoy!

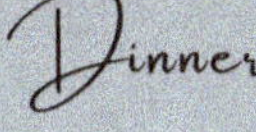

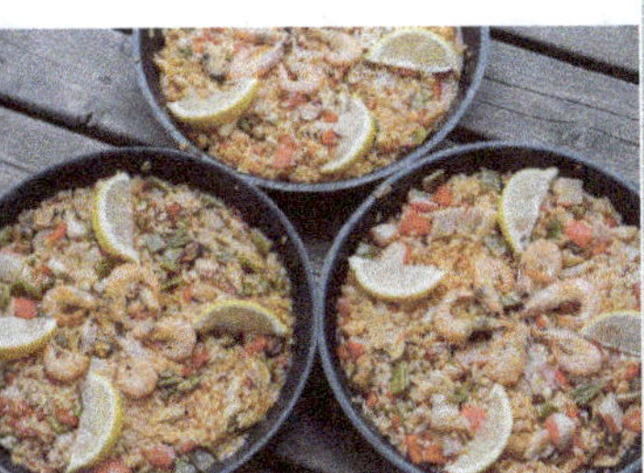

Lemon Garlic Shrimp with Cauliflower Rice
Ingredients:
- 4 oz. shrimp, peeled and deveined
- Juice of 1/2 lemon
- 1 clove garlic, minced
- 1 tsp olive oil
- 1 cup cauliflower rice
- Instructions: Marinate shrimp in lemon juice and garlic. Heat olive oil in a skillet and cook shrimp until pink and opaque. Serve over cooked cauliflower rice.

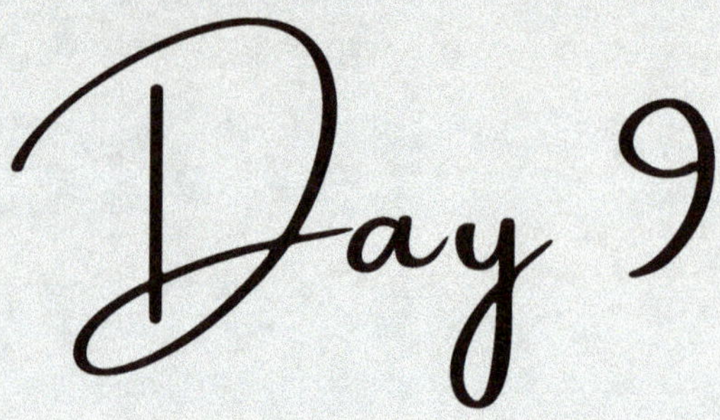

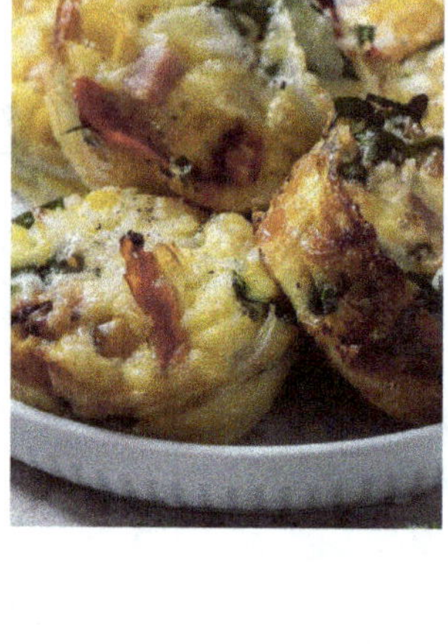

Veggie and Cheese Omelette Muffins
Ingredients:
- 4 eggs
- Diced bell peppers, onions, spinach
- Shredded cheese
- Instructions: Preheat oven to 350°F (175°C). In a bowl, whisk eggs and stir in diced vegetables and cheese. Pour mixture into greased muffin tins and bake for 20-25 minutes, or until set.

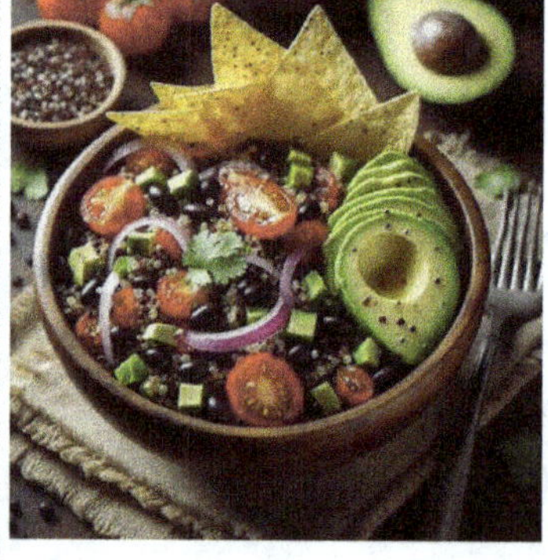

Quinoa and Black Bean Salad
Ingredients:
- Cooked quinoa
- Black beans, drained and rinsed
- Diced bell peppers, tomatoes, red onion
- Cilantro lime dressing
- Instructions: Combine all ingredients in a bowl and toss with dressing.

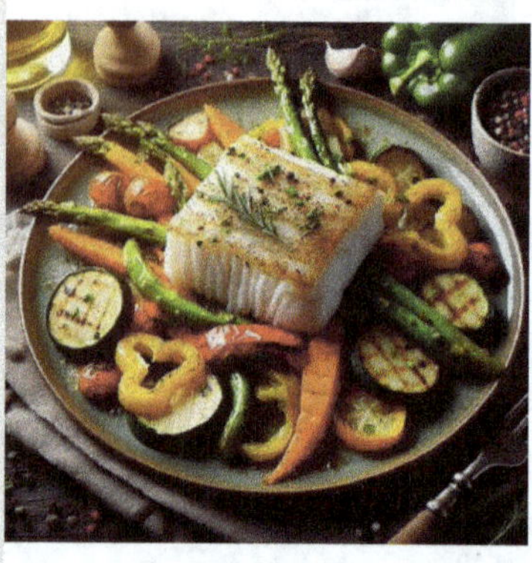

Baked Cod with Roasted Vegetables
Ingredients:
- 4 oz. cod fillet
- Lemon slices
- Mixed vegetables (zucchini, cherry
- tomatoes, bell peppers)
- Olive oil
- Instructions: Preheat oven to 400°F (200°C). Place cod fillet on a baking sheet, top with lemon slices, and drizzle with olive oil. Surround with mixed vegetables. Bake for 15-20 minutes, or until fish is cooked through and vegetables are tender.

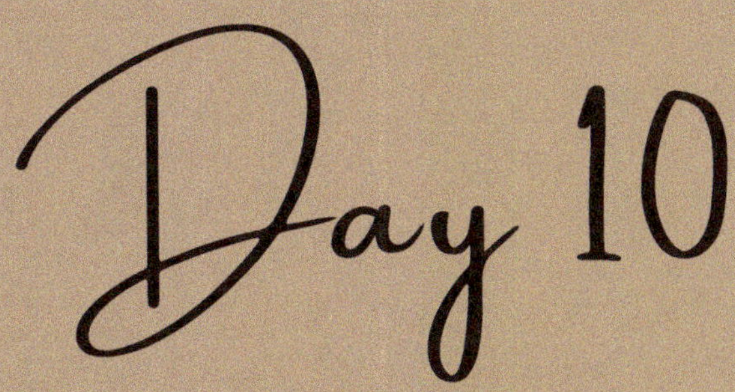

Breakfast

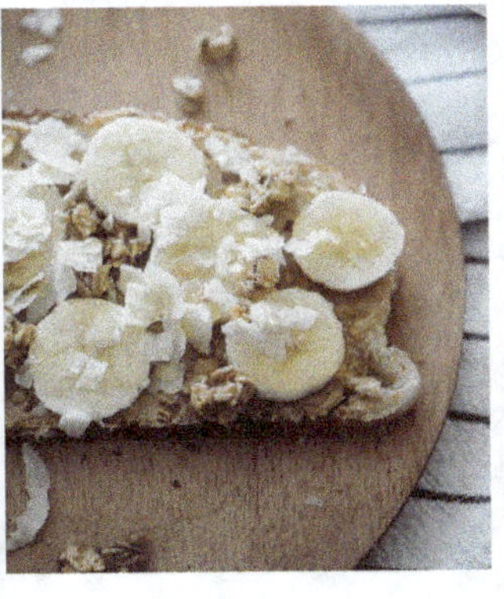

Peanut Butter Banana Overnight Oats
Ingredients:
- 1/2 cup rolled oats
- 1/2 cup almond milk
- 1 tbsp peanut butter
- 1/2 ripe banana, mashed
- Optional toppings: sliced banana, chopped nuts, drizzle of honey
- Instructions: In a jar or container, combine rolled oats, almond milk, peanut butter, and mashed banana. Stir well, cover, and refrigerate overnight. In the morning, stir again and add desired toppings before serving.

Lunch

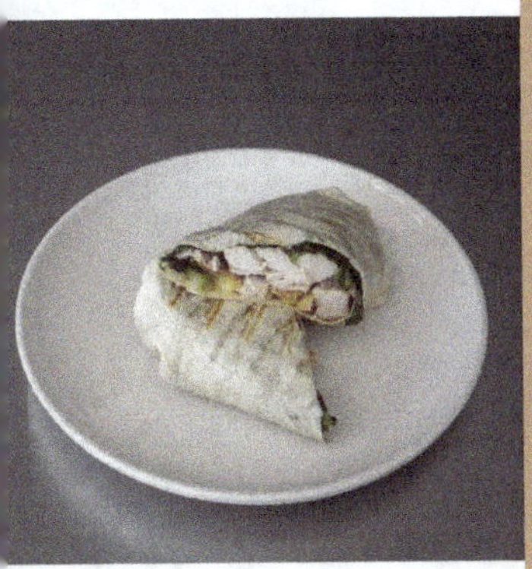

Turkey and Avocado Wrap
Ingredients:
- Whole wheat tortilla
- Sliced turkey breast
- Sliced avocado
- Mixed greens
- Dijon mustard or hummus
- Instructions: Spread mustard or hummus on tortilla. Layer with turkey slices, avocado, and mixed greens. Roll up tightly and cut in half.

Dinner

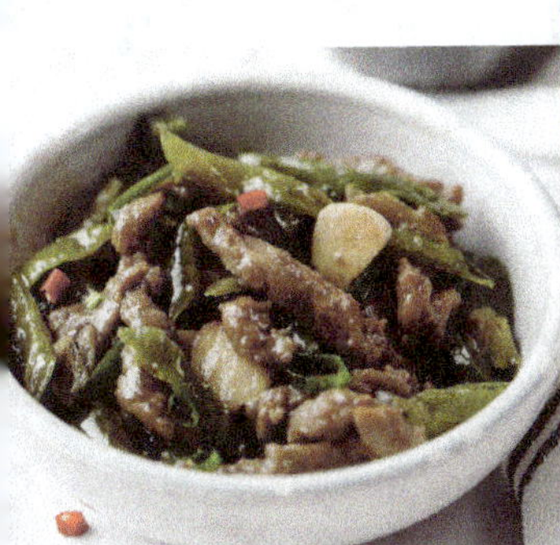

Beef and Broccoli Stir-Fry with Brown Rice
Ingredients:
- Thinly sliced beef steak
- Broccoli florets
- Low-sodium soy sauce
- Garlic, minced
- 1 cup cooked brown rice
- Instructions: Stir-fry beef and broccoli in garlic and soy sauce until beef is cooked through and broccoli is tender. Serve over cooked brown rice.

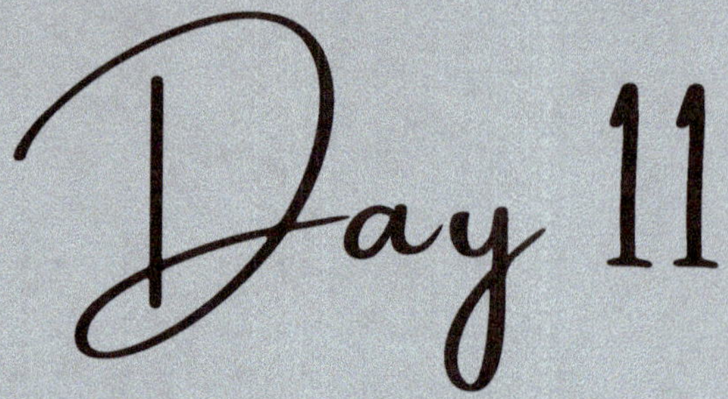

Day 11

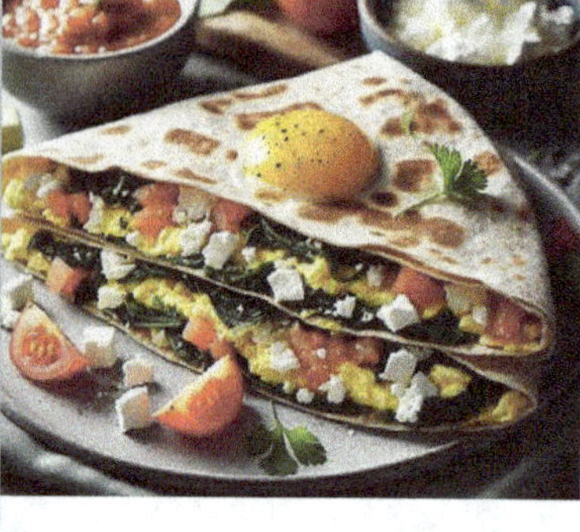

Spinach and Feta Breakfast Quesadilla
Ingredients:
- Whole wheat tortilla
- Handful of spinach leaves
- Crumbled feta cheese
- 1 egg, scrambled
- Instructions: Heat a skillet over medium heat. Place tortilla in the skillet and top with spinach, scrambled egg, and feta cheese. Fold the tortilla in half and cook until crispy on both sides.

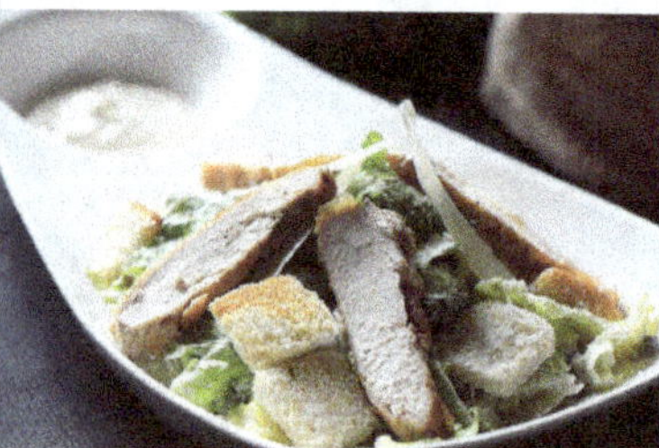

Chicken Caesar Salad
Ingredients:
- Grilled chicken breast, sliced
- Romaine lettuce
- Cherry tomatoes, halved
- Shaved Parmesan cheese
- Caesar dressing
- Instructions: Toss together all ingredients in a bowl with Caesar dressing.

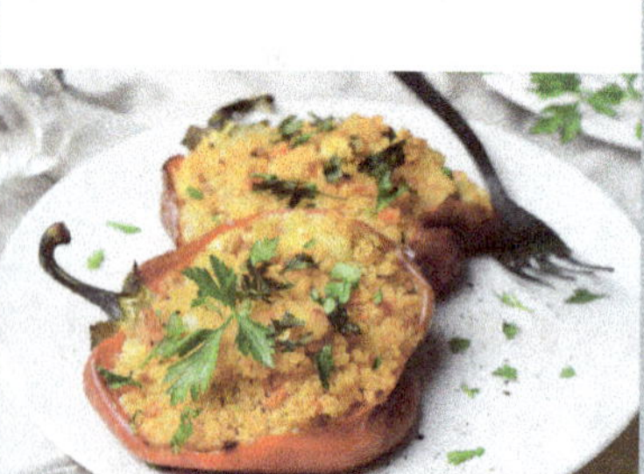

Turkey and Vegetable Stuffed Bell Peppers
Ingredients:
- Bell peppers, halved and seeded
- Lean ground turkey
- Chopped onion, zucchini, and mushrooms
- Cooked quinoa
- Marinara sauce
- Instructions: Preheat oven to 375°F (190°C). In a skillet, cook ground turkey with chopped vegetables until browned. Stir in cooked quinoa and marinara sauce. Spoon mixture into halved bell peppers and bake for 25-30 minutes, or until peppers are tender.

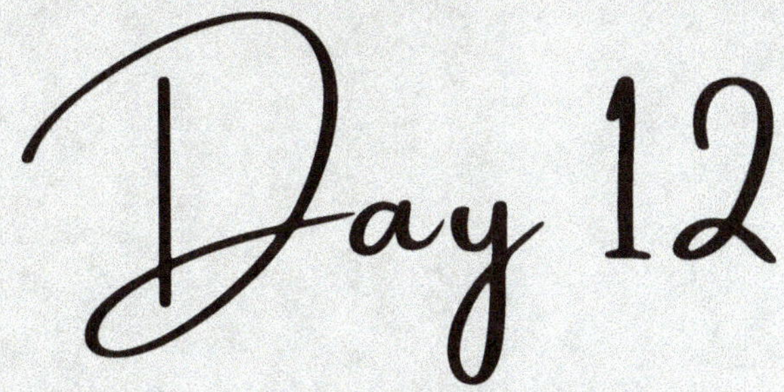

Day 12

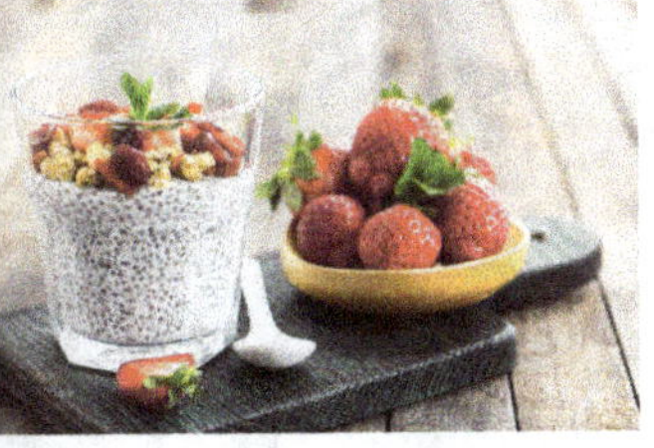

Berry Chia Seed Pudding
Ingredients:
- 1/4 cup chia seeds
- 1 cup almond milk
- Mixed berries
- Optional sweetener (honey, maple syrup)
- Instructions: Mix chia seeds and almond milk in a jar or bowl. Let sit in the fridge for at least 2 hours or overnight, until thickened. Serve with mixed berries on top.

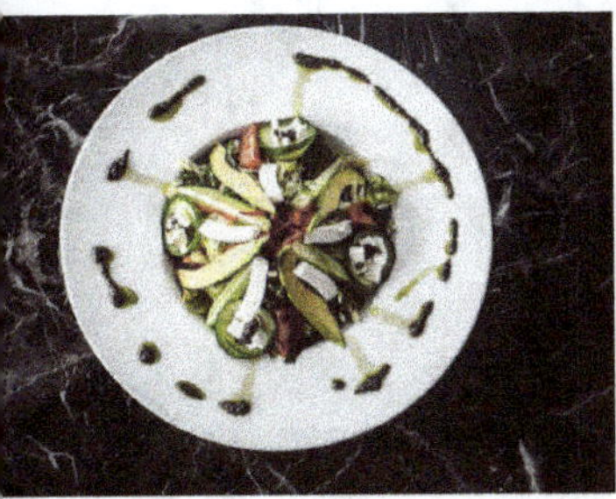

Turkey and Avocado Salad
Ingredients:
- Mixed greens
- Sliced turkey breast
- Sliced avocado
- Cherry tomatoes, halved
- Balsamic vinaigrette dressing
- Instructions: Toss together all ingredients in bowl with balsamic vinaigrette dressing.

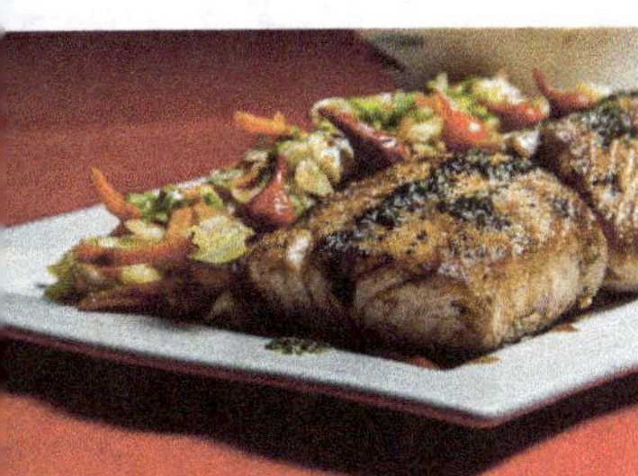

Baked Salmon with Roasted Vegetables
Ingredients:
- Salmon fillets
- Assorted vegetables (such as carrots,
- broccoli, and cauliflower)
- Olive oil
- Lemon slices
- Instructions: Preheat oven to 400°F (200°C). Place salmon fillets on a baking sheet lined with parchment paper. Arrange vegetables around the salmon. Drizzle everything with olive oil and season with salt, pepper, and lemon slices. Bake for 15-20 minutes, or until salmon is cooked through and vegetables are tender.

Day 13

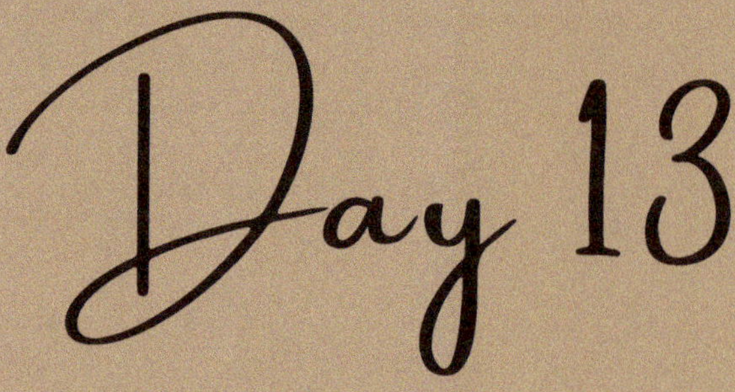

Banana Nut Overnight Oats
Ingredients:
- 1/2 cup rolled oats
- 1/2 cup almond milk
- 1/2 ripe banana, mashed
- 1 tbsp chopped nuts (such as almonds or walnuts
- Instructions: Mix rolled oats, almond milk, mashed banana, and chopped nuts in a jar or container. Stir well, cover, and refrigerate overnight. Enjoy cold in the morning.

Lunch

Veggie and Hummus Wrap
Ingredients:
- Whole wheat tortilla
- Hummus
- Sliced cucumber, bell pepper, and avocado
- Mixed greens
- Instructions: Spread hummus on tortilla. Layer with sliced vegetables and mixed greens. Roll up tightly and slice in half.

Dinner

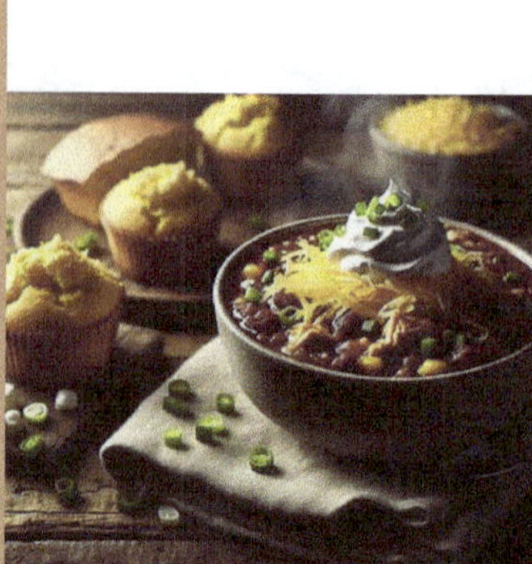

Turkey Chili with Cornbread Muffins
Ingredients:
- Ground turkey
- Diced onion, bell pepper, and tomatoes
- Kidney beans, drained and rinsed
- Tomato sauce
- Chili powder, cumin, garlic powder
- Cornbread mix
- Instructions: In a large pot, cook ground turkey with diced vegetables until browned. Add kidney beans, tomato sauce, and spices. Simmer for 20-30 minutes. Meanwhile, prepare cornbread muffins according to package instructions. Serve chili with cornbread muffins on the side.

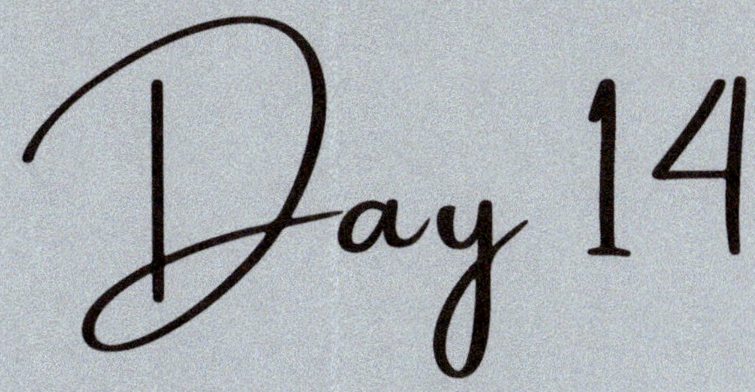

Day 14

Berry Blast Smoothie Bowl
Ingredients:
- 1/2 cup frozen mixed berries
- 1/2 ripe banana
- 1/4 cup Greek yogurt
- 1/4 cup almond milk
- Toppings: sliced strawberries, granola, chia
- seeds
- Instructions: Blend frozen berries, banana, Greek yogurt, and almond milk until smooth. Pour into a bowl and top with sliced strawberries, granola, and chia seeds.

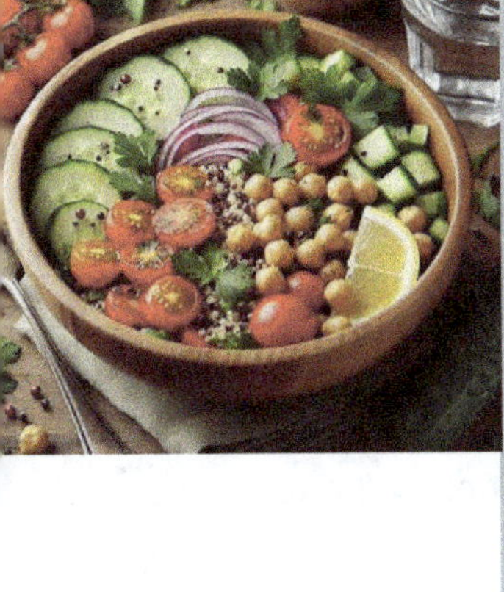

Quinoa and Chickpea Salad
Ingredients:
- Cooked quinoa
- Cooked chickpeas, drained and rinsed
- Diced cucumber, cherry tomatoes, and red
- onion
- Chopped fresh parsley
- Lemon tahini dressing
- Instructions: Combine all ingredients in a bowl and toss with lemon tahini dressing.

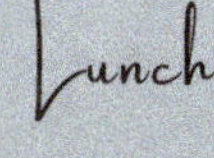
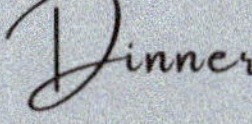

Lemon Garlic Salmon with Steamed Broccoli and Sweet Potato
Ingredients:
- Salmon fillets
- Lemon juice and zest
- Minced garlic
- Olive oil
- Steamed broccoli
- Baked sweet potato
- Instructions: Marinate salmon in lemon juice,
- zest, minced garlic, and olive oil. Bake until cooked through. Serve with steamed broccoli and baked sweet potato

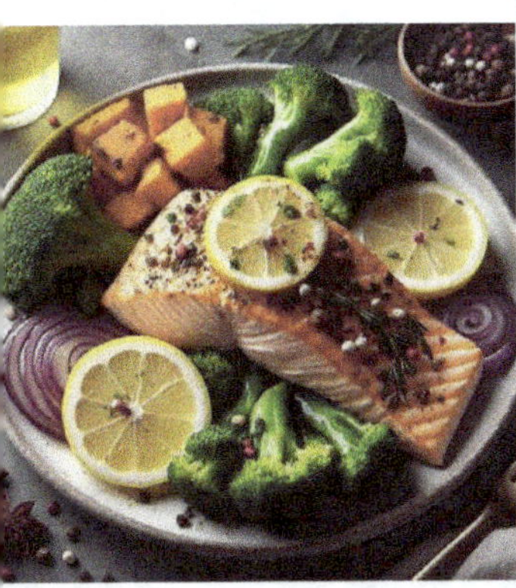

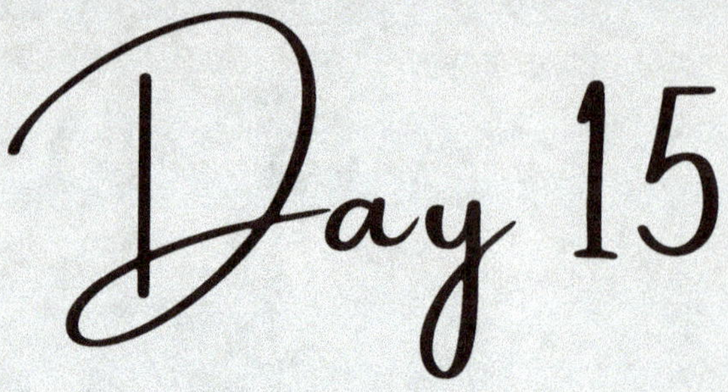

Day 15

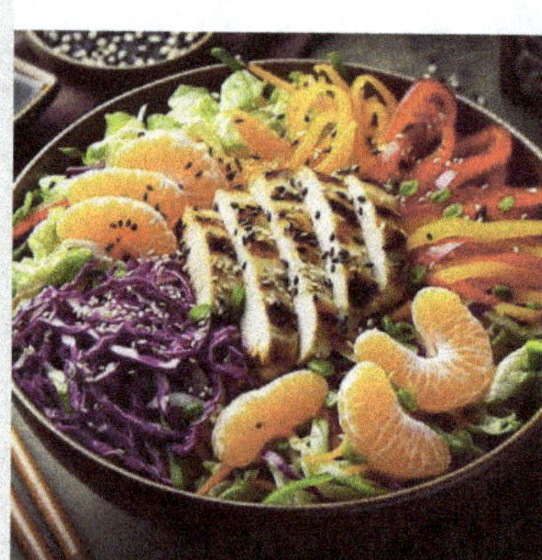

Sweet Potato Hash with Eggs
Ingredients:

- Sweet potatoes
- Eggs
- Sautéed bell peppers and onions
- Olive oil
- Salt, pepper
- Instructions: Dice sweet potatoes, bell peppers, and onion. Sauté in olive oil until tender. Create wells in the hash and crack eggs into them. Cover and cook until eggs are set. Season with salt and pepper.

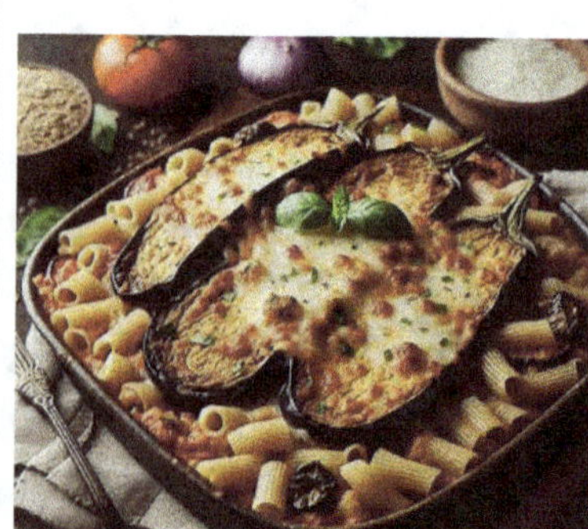

Asian-Inspired Chicken Salad
Ingredients:

- Grilled chicken breast, sliced.
- Mixed greens
- Mandarin orange
- Sliced almonds,
- Sesame dressing
- Instructions: Toss mixed greens with mandarin oranges, sliced almonds, and grilled chicken breast. Drizzle with sesame dressing and toss to combine.

Baked Eggplant Parmesan with Whole Wheat Pasta
Ingredients:

- Eggplant
- marinara sauce
- mozzarella cheese
- Parmesan cheese
- whole wheat pasta
- olive oil
- breadcrumbs
- Italian seasoning
- Instructions: Slice eggplant and coat with olive oil, breadcrumbs, and Italian seasoning. Bake until golden brown. Layer baked eggplant slices with marinara sauce and mozzarella cheese. Bake until cheese is melted and bubbly. Serve with cooked whole wheat pasta.

Day 16

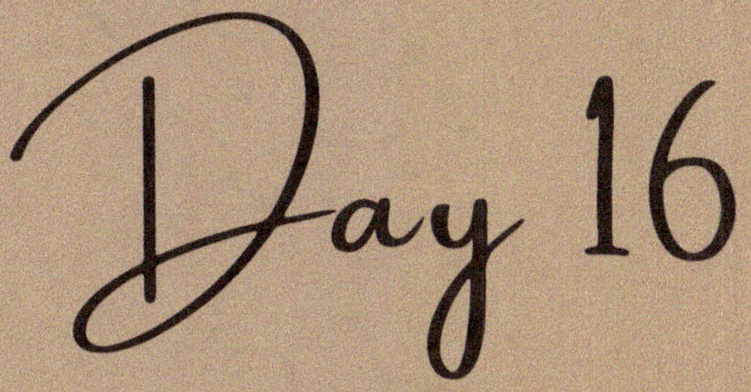

Breakfast

Spinach and Mushroom Egg Muffins
Ingredients:

- 4 eggs
- Handful of spinach leaves
- Sliced mushrooms
- Shredded cheese (optional)
- Instructions: Preheat oven to 350°F (175°C). In a bowl, whisk eggs and stir in spinach, mushrooms, and cheese. Pour mixture into greased muffin tins and bake for 20-25 minutes, or until set.

Lunch

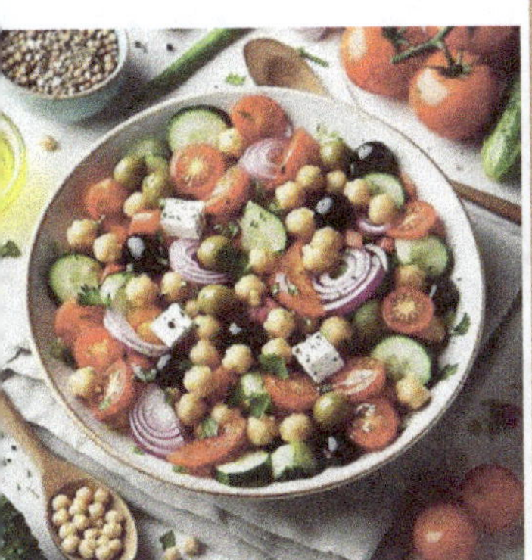

Mediterranean Chickpea Salad
Ingredients:

- Cooked quinoa
- Cooked chickpeas, drained and rinsed
- Diced cucumber, cherry tomatoes, and red onion
- Kalamata olives, sliced
- Crumbled feta cheese
- Lemon vinaigrette dressing
- Instructions: Toss together all ingredients in a bowl with lemon vinaigrette dressing.

Dinner

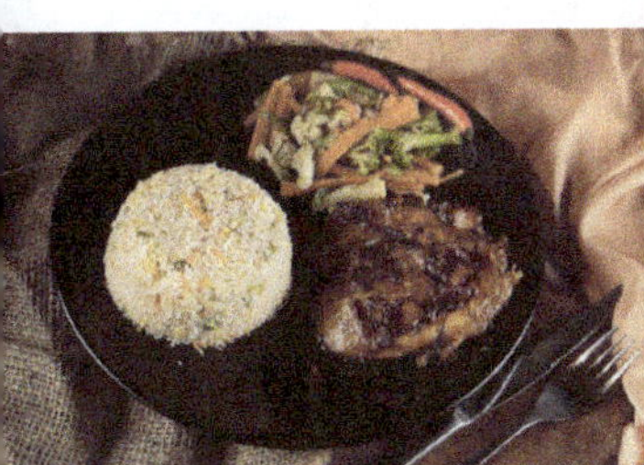

Turkey and Vegetable Stir-Fry with Cauliflower Rice
Ingredients:

- Lean ground turkey
- Stir-fry vegetables (such as bell peppers, snap peas, and carrots)
- Low-sodium stir-fry sauce
- Cooked cauliflower rice
- Instructions: Stir-fry ground turkey and vegetables in a skillet with stir-fry sauce until heated through. Serve over cooked cauliflower rice.

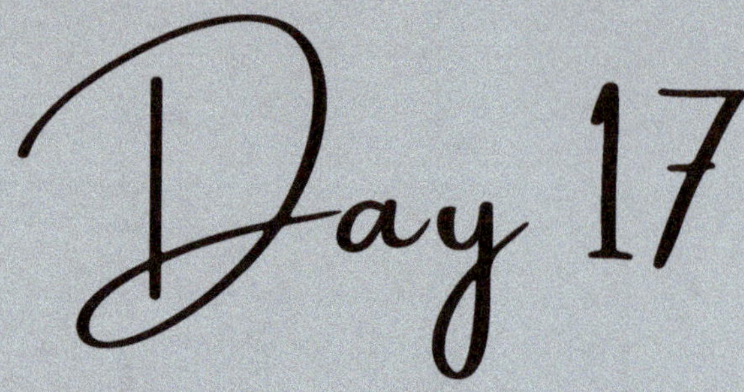

Day 17

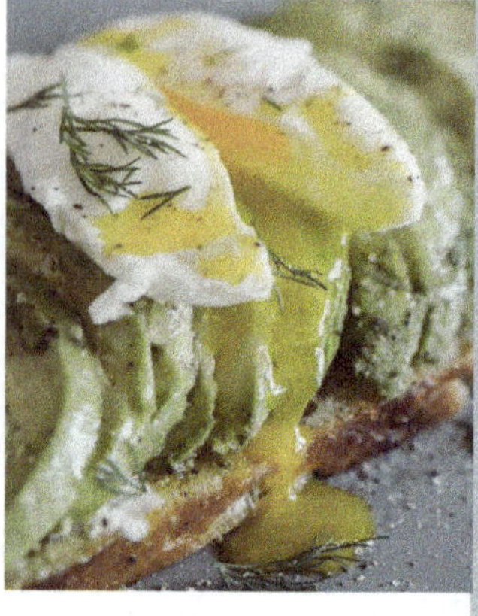

Avocado and Tomato Toast with Poached Egg
Ingredients:

- Whole grain bread
- Ripe avocado
- Sliced tomato
- Poached egg
- Instructions: Toast whole grain bread and top with mashed avocado, sliced tomato, and a poached egg.

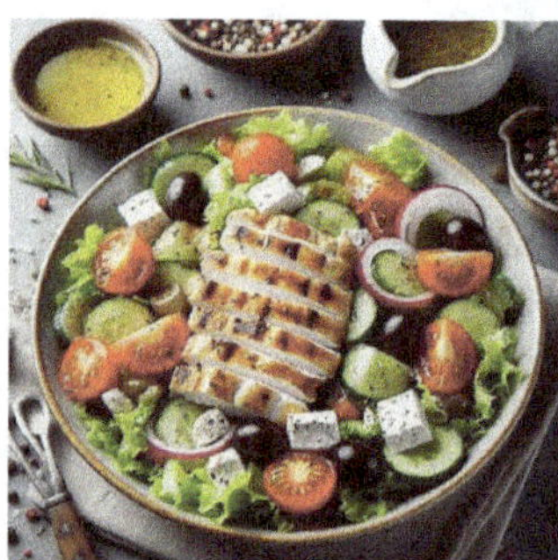

Greek Salad with Grilled Chicken
Ingredients:

- Mixed greens
- Grilled chicken breast, sliced
- Diced cucumber, cherry tomatoes, and red onion
- Kalamata olives
- Crumbled feta cheese
- Greek dressing
- Instructions: Toss together all ingredients in a bowl with Greek dressing.

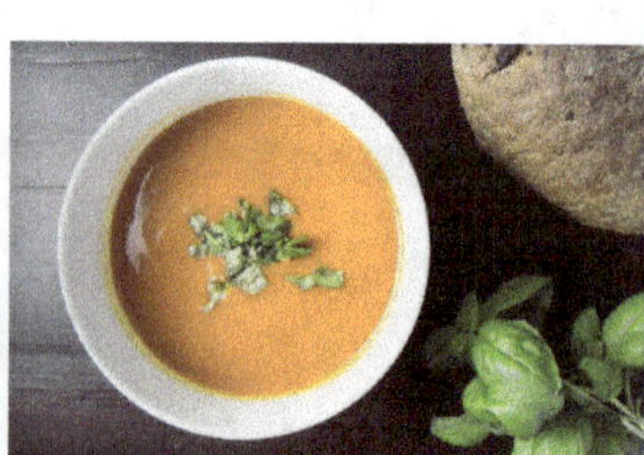

Veggie and Lentil Soup with Whole Grain Bread
Ingredients:

- Mixed vegetables (such as carrots,
- celery, and kale)
- Cooked lentils
- Low-sodium vegetable broth
- Herbs and spices (such as thyme,
- rosemary, and garlic powder)
- Instructions: Combine all ingredients in a pot and simmer until vegetables are tender. Serve with whole grain bread on the side.

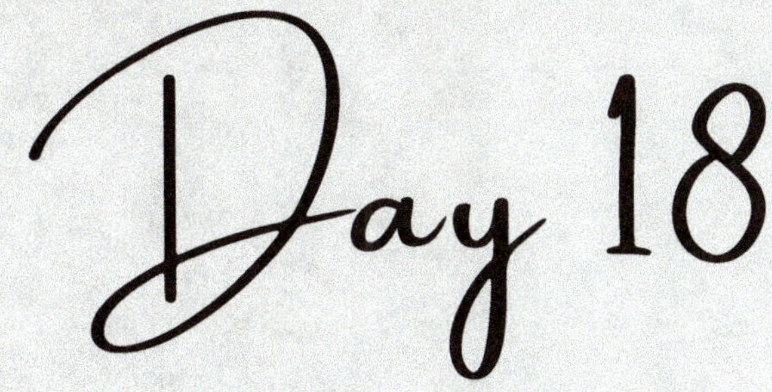

Day 18

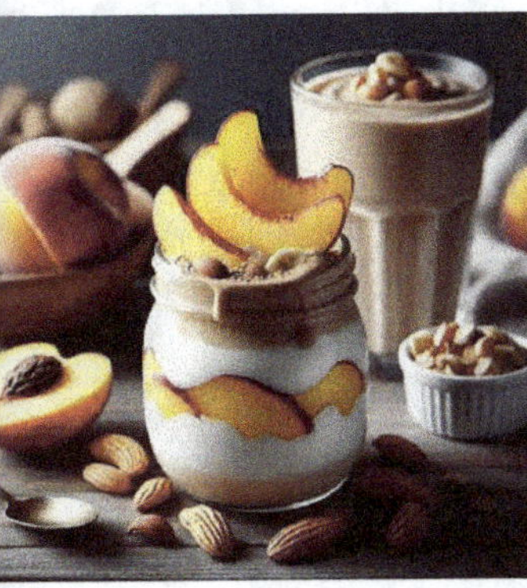

Breakfast

Peach Yogurt Parfait
Ingredients:
- Greek yogurt
- Sliced almonds
- Peaches
- Instructions: Layer Greek yogurt, sliced peaches, and almonds in a glass or bowl.

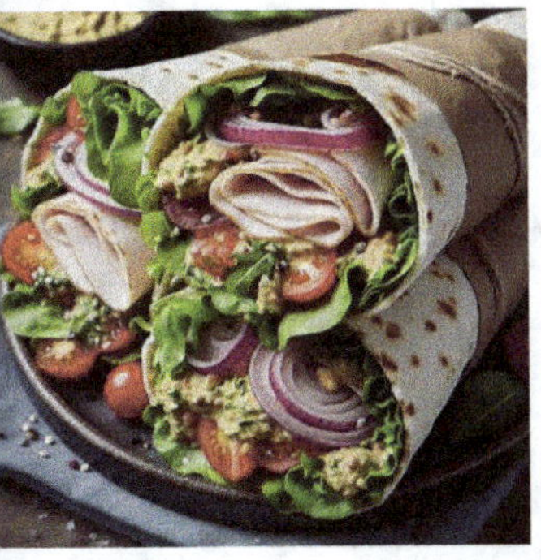

Lunch

Turkey and Hummus Wrap with Mixed Greens
Ingredients:
- Whole wheat tortilla
- Sliced turkey breast
- Hummus
- Mixed greens
- Instructions: Spread hummus on tortilla. Layer with turkey slices and mixed greens. Roll up tightly and slice in half.

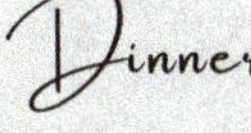

Dinner

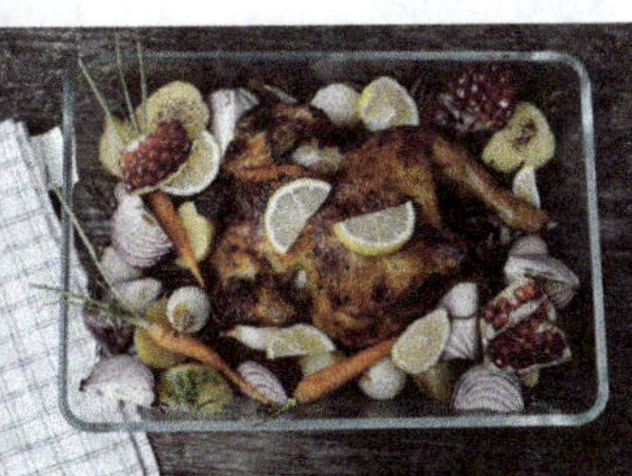

Lemon Herb Grilled Chicken with Roasted Vegetables
Ingredients:
- Chicken breast
- Lemon juice and zest
- Mixed herbs (such as rosemary, thyme, and oregano)
- Assorted vegetables (such as bell peppers, zucchini, and cherry tomatoes)
- Instructions: Marinate chicken in lemon juice, zest, and herbs. Grill until cooked through. Serve with roasted vegetables.

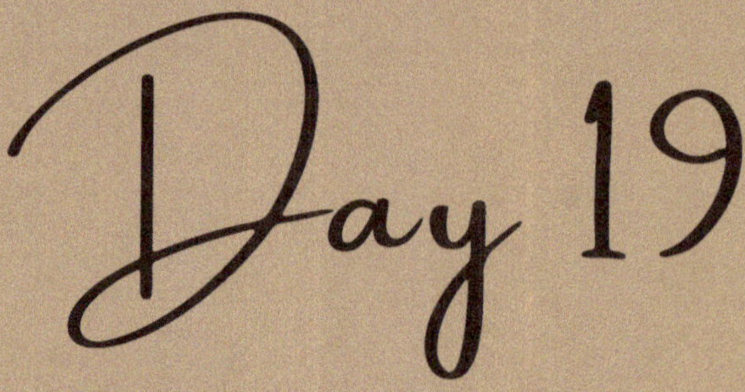

Day 19

Breakfast

Blueberry Almond Smoothie Bowl
Ingredients:
- 1/2 cup frozen blueberries
- 1/2 ripe banana
- 1/4 cup Greek yogurt
- 1/4 cup almond milk
- Toppings: sliced almonds, fresh blueberries,
- granola
- Instructions: Blend frozen blueberries, banana, Greek yogurt, and almond milk until smooth. Pour into a bowl and top with sliced almonds, fresh blueberries, and granola.

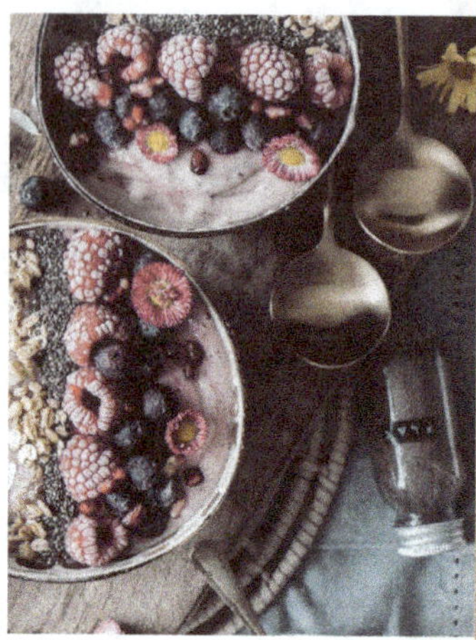

Lunch

Quinoa and Black Bean Stuffed Bell Peppers
Ingredients:
- Bell peppers, halved and seeded
- Cooked quinoa
- Black beans, drained and rinsed
- Diced tomatoes, corn, and red onion
- Shredded cheese
- Instructions: Preheat oven to 375°F (190°C). In a bowl, mix cooked quinoa, black beans, diced tomatoes, corn, and red onion. Stuff mixture into halved bell peppers. Top with shredded cheese. Bake for 20-25 minutes, or until peppers are tender.

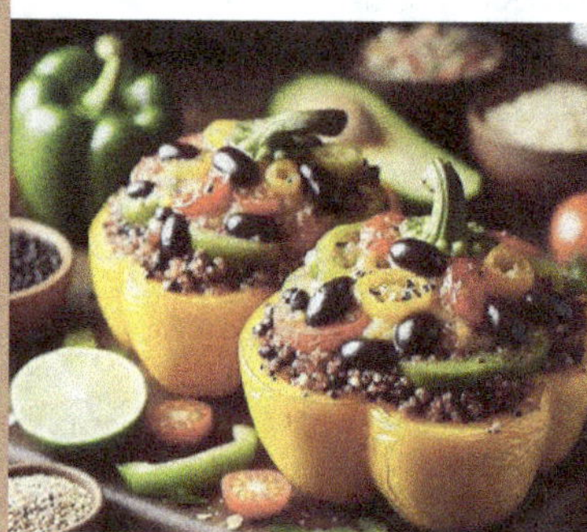

Dinner

Shrimp and Vegetable Stir-Fry with Brown Rice
Ingredients:
- Shrimp, peeled and deveined
- Stir-fry vegetables (such as broccoli, bell
- peppers, and snap peas)
- Low-sodium stir-fry sauce
- Cooked brown rice
- Instructions: Stir-fry shrimp and vegetables in a skillet with stir-fry sauce until shrimp is pink and vegetables are tender. Serve over cooked brown rice.

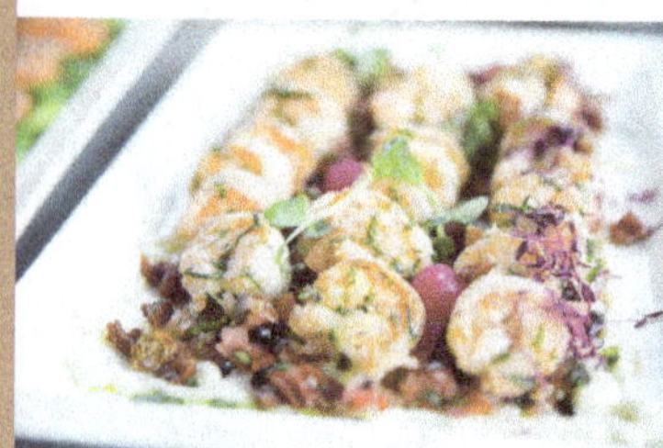

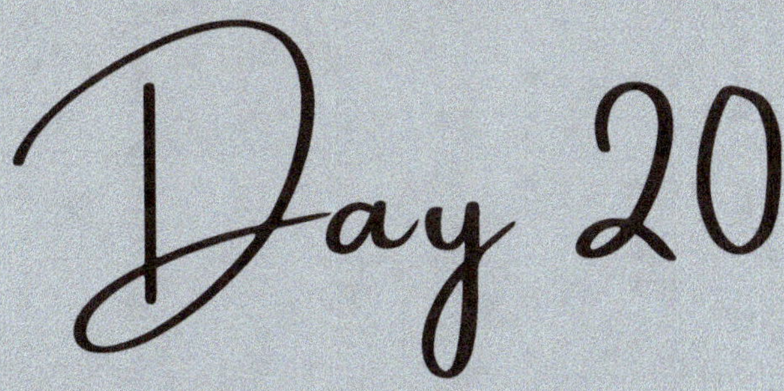

Day 20

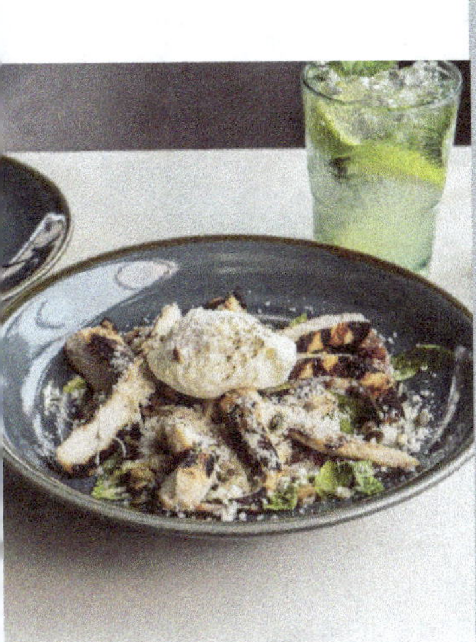

Spinach and Feta Breakfast Quesadilla
Ingredients:

- Whole wheat tortilla
- Handful of spinach leaves
- Crumbled feta cheese
- 1 egg, scrambled
- Instructions: Heat a skillet over medium heat. Place tortilla in the skillet and top with spinach, scrambled egg, and feta cheese. Fold the tortilla in half and cook until crispy on both sides.

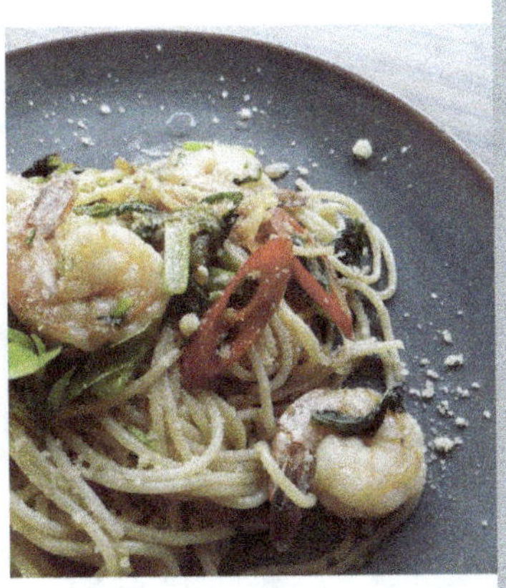
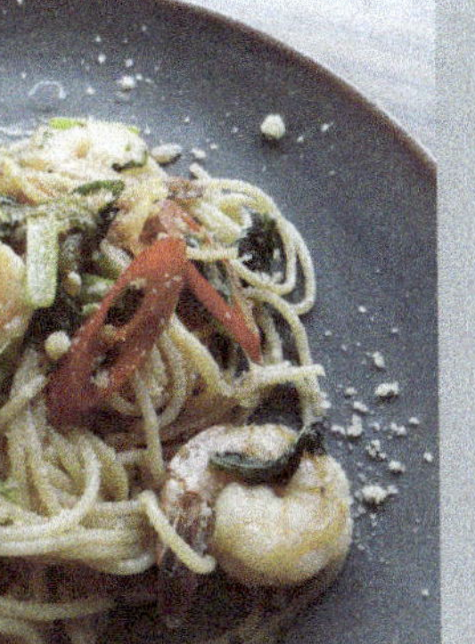

Grilled Chicken Salad
Ingredients:

- Chicken breast
- Mixed greens
- Cucumber
- Crumbled goat cheese
- Balsamic vinaigrette dressing
- Instructions: Grill chicken breast until cooked through. Toss mixed greens and cucumber with balsamic vinaigrette. Top with sliced grilled chicken.

Lemon Garlic Shrimp with Zucchini Noodles
Ingredients:

- Shrimp
- Zucchini, spiralized into noodles
- Minced garlic
- Lemon juice
- Olive oil
- Instructions: Sauté shrimp in olive oil with minced garlic until pink. Add lemon juice and zucchini noodles, then cook until noodles are tender. Serve hot.

Day 21

Breakfast

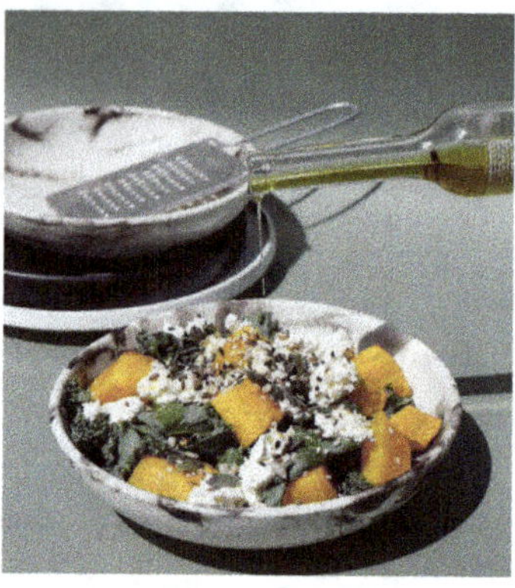

Cottage Cheese and Pineapple Bowl
Ingredients:
- Cottage cheese
- Fresh pineapple chunks
- Instructions: Serve cottage cheese topped with fresh pineapple chunks.

Lunch

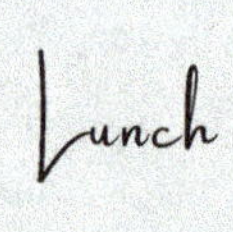
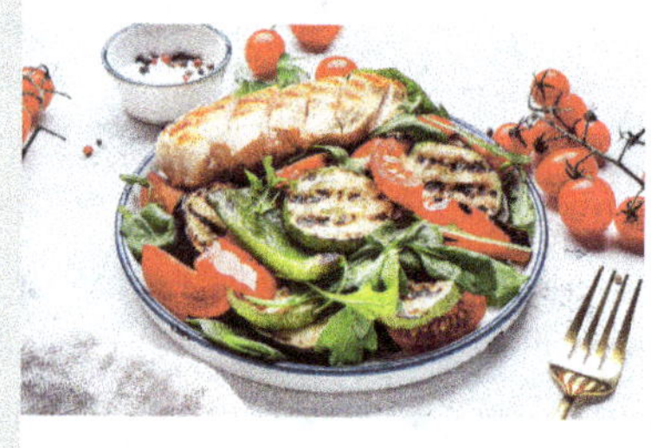

Turkey and Hummus Wrap with Mixed Greens
Ingredients:
- Whole wheat tortilla
- Sliced turkey breast
- Hummus
- Mixed greens
- Instructions: Spread hummus on tortilla. Layer with turkey slices and mixed greens. Roll up tightly and slice in half.

Dinner

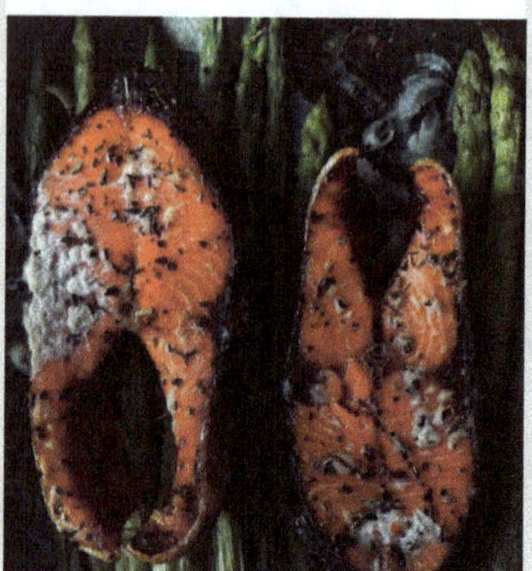

Baked Salmon with Roasted Asparagus and Quinoa
Ingredients:
- Salmon fillet
- Asparagus
- Quinoa
- Olive oil
- Lemon
- Salt & pepper
- Instructions: Marinate chicken in lemon juice, zest, and herbs. Grill until cooked through. Serve with roasted vegetables.

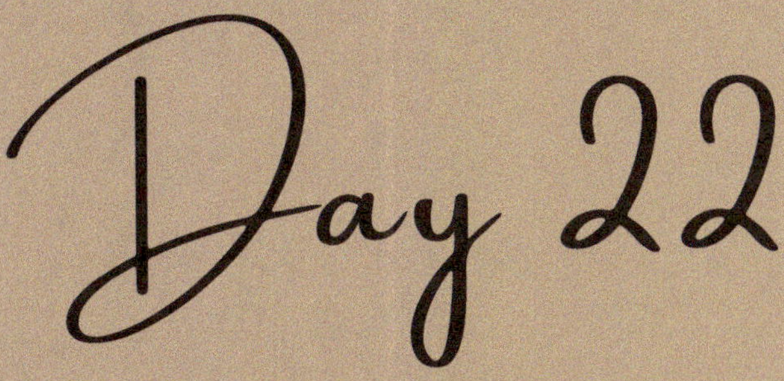

Day 22

Protein-Packed Pancakes
Ingredients:
- Protein pancake mix
- Sliced peaches
- Sliced almonds,
- Maple syrup
- Instructions: Prepare protein pancake mix according to package instructions. Cook pancakes on a griddle until golden brown. Serve topped with sliced peaches, sliced almonds, and a drizzle of maple syrup.

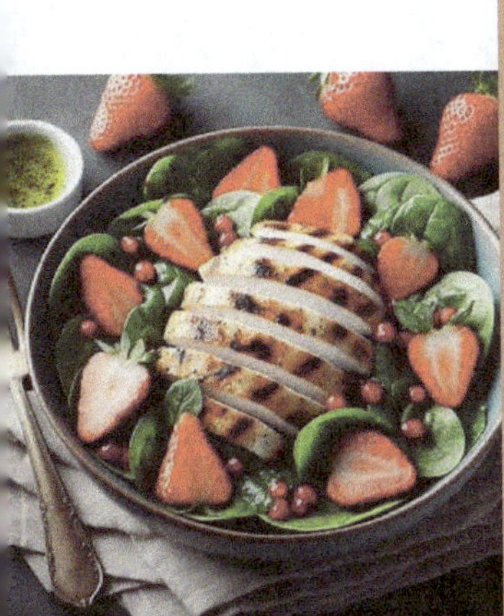

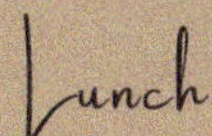

Spinach and Strawberry Salad with Grilled Chicken
Ingredients:
- Baby spinach
- Sliced strawberries
- Sliced almonds
- Grilled chicken breast
- Balsamic vinaigrette
- Instructions: Toss baby spinach with sliced strawberries, sliced almonds, and grilled chicken breast. Drizzle with balsamic vinaigrette and toss to combine.

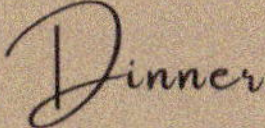

Lemon Garlic Salmon with Steamed Broccoli and Sweet Potato
Ingredients:
- Salmon fillets
- Lemon juice and zest
- Minced garlic
- Olive oil
- Steamed broccoli
- Baked sweet potato
- Instructions: Marinate salmon in lemon juice, zest, minced garlic, and olive oil. Bake until cooked through. Serve with steamed broccoli and baked sweet potato.

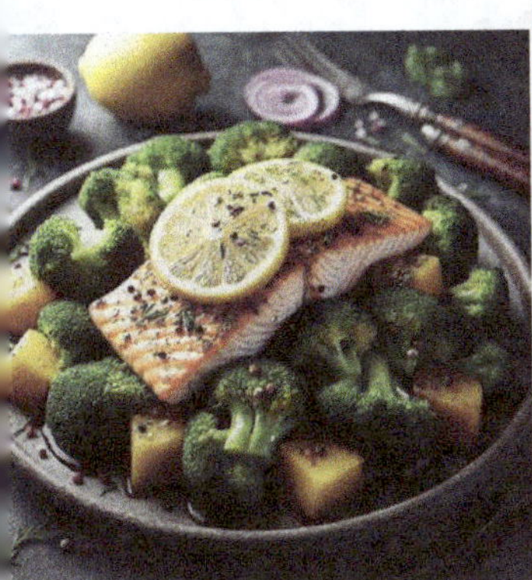

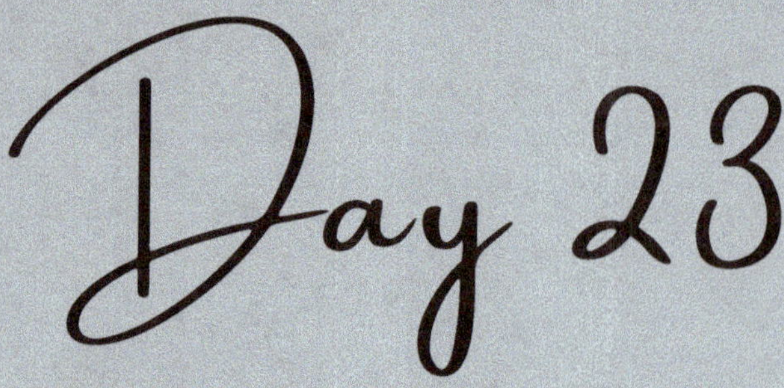

Day 23

Veggie Omelette with Whole Grain Toast
Ingredients:

- 2 eggs
- Diced bell peppers, onions, spinach
- Shredded cheese (optional)
- Whole grain toast
- Instructions: In a skillet, cook diced vegetables until tender. Pour beaten eggs over the vegetables and cook until set. Sprinkle with shredded cheese if desired. Serve with whole grain toast.

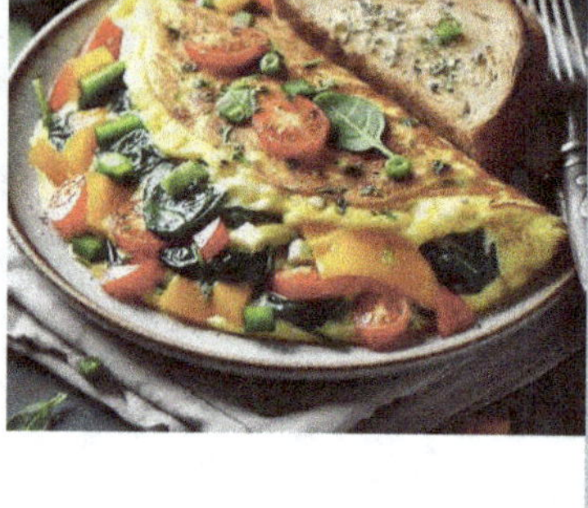

Grilled Chicken Salad with Strawberries and Almonds
Ingredients:

- Mixed greens
- Grilled chicken breast, sliced
- Sliced strawberries
- Sliced almonds
- Balsamic vinaigrette dressing
- Instructions: Toss together all ingredients in a bowl with balsamic vinaigrette dressing.

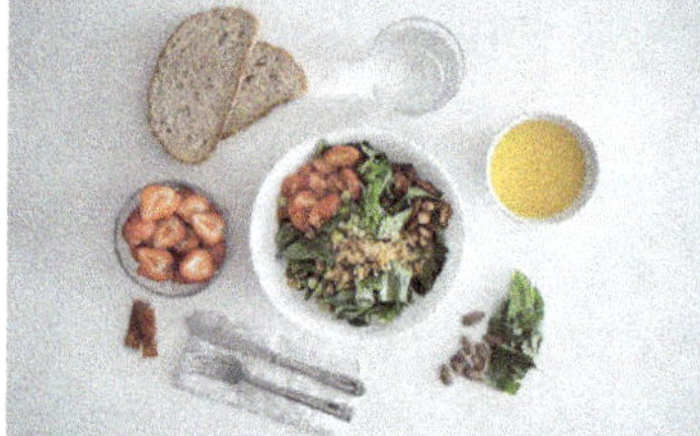

Lentil and Vegetable Curry with Brown Rice
Ingredients:

- Cooked lentils
- Mixed vegetables (such as carrots,
- cauliflower, and bell peppers)
- Curry paste or powder
- Coconut milk
- Cooked brown rice
- Instructions: In a pot, sauté mixed vegetables until tender. Add cooked lentils, curry paste or powder, and coconut milk. Simmer until flavors are well combined. Serve over cooked brown rice

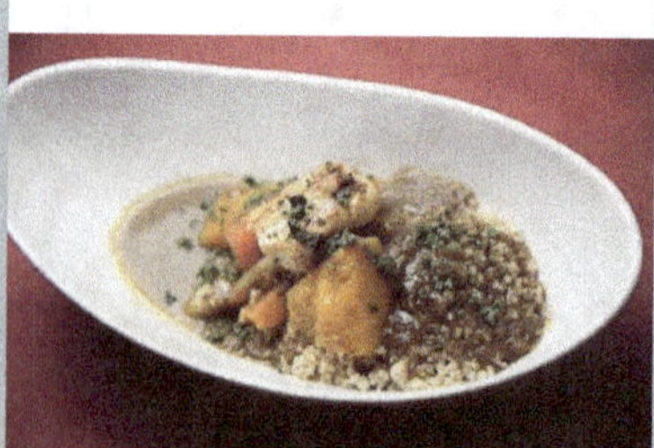

Day 24

Mediterranean Egg Wrap
Ingredients:
- Whole wheat tortilla
- Scrambled eggs
- Diced tomatoes
- Chopped olives
- Crumbled feta cheese
- Fresh basil
- Instructions: Fill a whole wheat tortilla with scrambled eggs, diced tomatoes, chopped olives, crumbled feta cheese, and fresh basil. Roll up and serve

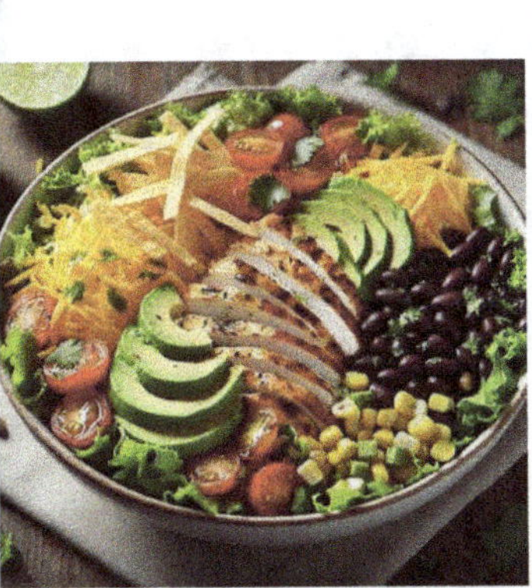

Southwest Chicken Salad
Ingredients:
- Grilled chicken breast
- mixed greens
- corn
- black beans
- cherry tomatoes
- avocado
- shredded cheese
- tortilla strips
- ranch dressing
- Instructions: Toss mixed greens with grilled chicken breast, corn, black beans, halved cherry tomatoes, diced avocado, shredded cheese, and tortilla strips. Drizzle with ranch dressing.

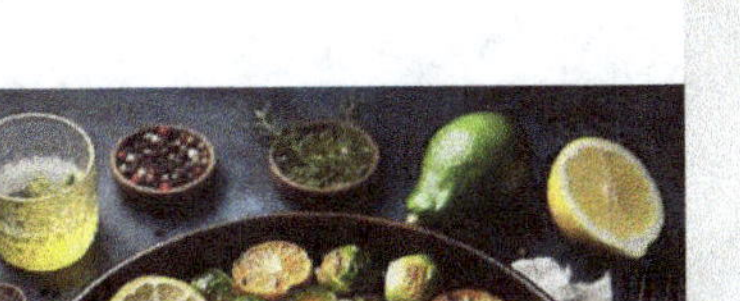

Baked Cod with Lemon and Herbs, Served with Roasted Brussels Sprouts
Ingredients:
- Cod fillets
- Lemon slices
- Mixed herbs (such as parsley, thyme, and
- dill)
- Olive oil
- Brussels sprouts
- Instructions: Preheat oven to 400°F (200°C). Place cod fillets on a baking sheet lined with parchment paper. Top with lemon slices, mixed herbs, and a drizzle of olive oil. Bake for 15-20 minutes, or until fish is cooked through. Serve with roasted Brussels sprouts.

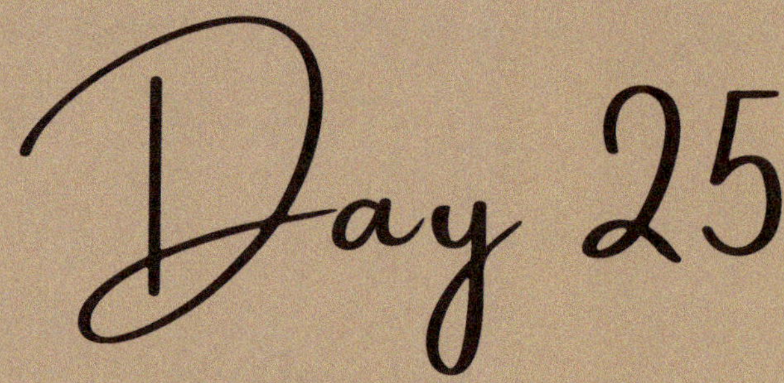

Spinach and Mushroom Omelette
Ingredients:
- 2 eggs
- Handful of spinach
- Sliced mushrooms
- Salt and pepper to taste
- Instructions: Beat eggs in a bowl. Heat a non-stick skillet over medium heat, add spinach and mushrooms, then pour in beaten eggs. Cook until set, fold in half, and serve.

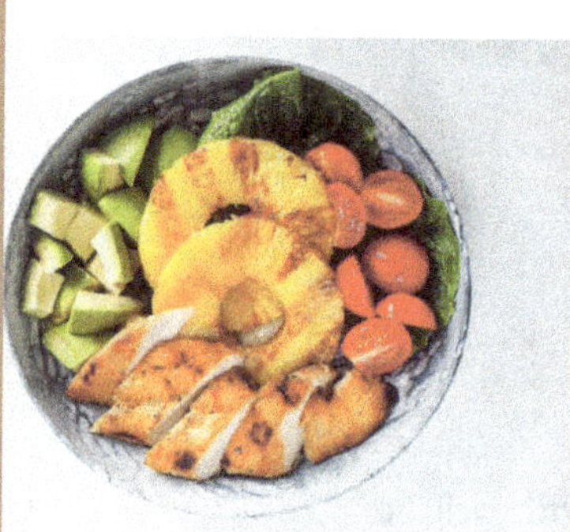

Grilled Chicken Salad with Avocado
Ingredients:
- Grilled chicken breast
- Mixed greens
- Sliced avocado
- Cherry tomatoes
- Balsamic vinaigrette dressing
- Instructions: Toss all ingredients together in a bowl and drizzle with balsamic vinaigrette dressing.

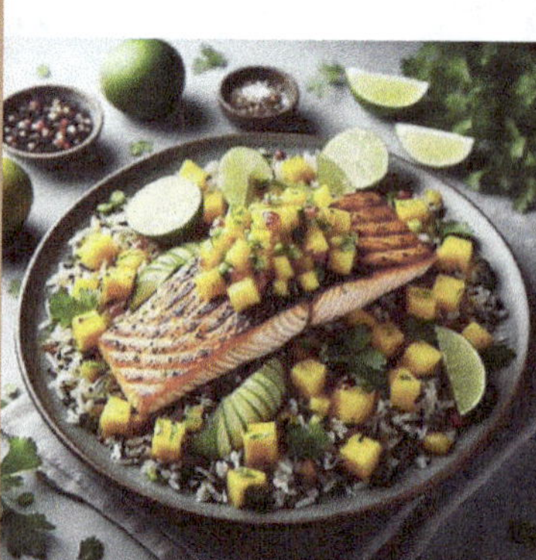

Grilled Salmon with Mango Salsa
Ingredients:
- Salmon fillet
- Lime juice
- Mango
- Red onion
- Jalapeño
- Cilantro
- Garlic powder
- Salt and pepper to taste
- Olive oil
- Instructions: Season salmon fillets with olive oil, salt, and pepper. Grill until cooked through. Dice mango, red onion, and jalapeño. Mix with chopped cilantro and lime juice to make salsa. Serve grilled salmon with mango salsa on top.

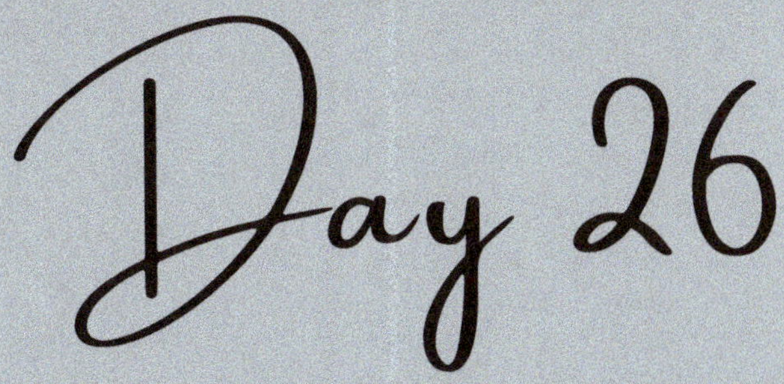

Day 26

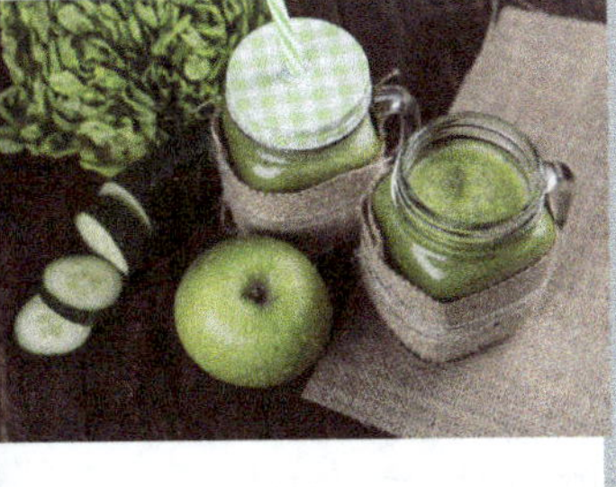

Green Smoothie with Spinach and Pineapple
Ingredients:
- Handful of spinach
- 1/2 cup frozen pineapple
- 1/2 banana
- 1/2 cup unsweetened almond milk
- Instructions: Blend all ingredients until smooth. Add more almond milk if needed for desired consistency.

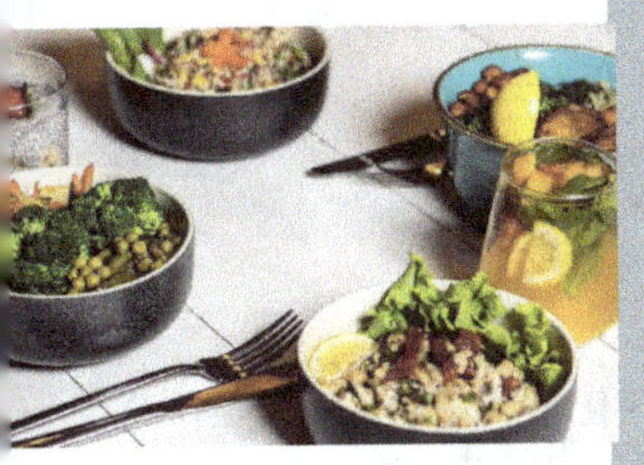

Chicken and Vegetable Salad with Citrus Dressing
Ingredients:
- Grilled chicken breast
- Mixed greens
- Sliced bell peppers
- Sliced oranges
- Citrus vinaigrette dressing
- Instructions: Arrange all ingredients on a plate and drizzle with citrus vinaigrette dressing.

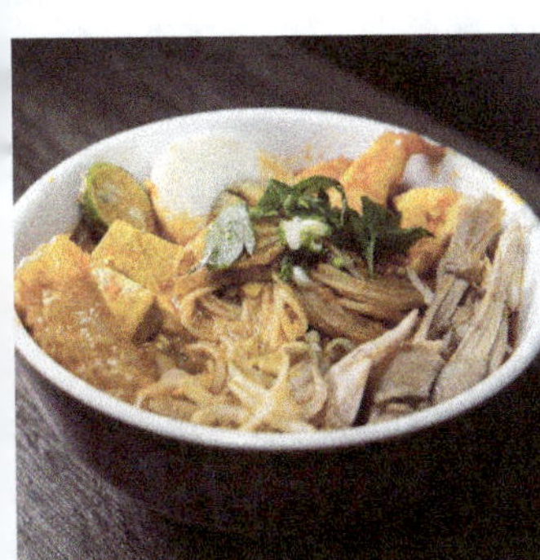

Spicy Shrimp with Zucchini Noodles
Ingredients:
- Shrimp
- Zucchini, spiralized into noodles
- Crushed red pepper flakes
- Garlic
- Olive oil
- Instructions: Sauté shrimp in olive oil with minced garlic and crushed red pepper flakes. Add zucchini noodles and cook until tender. Serve hot.

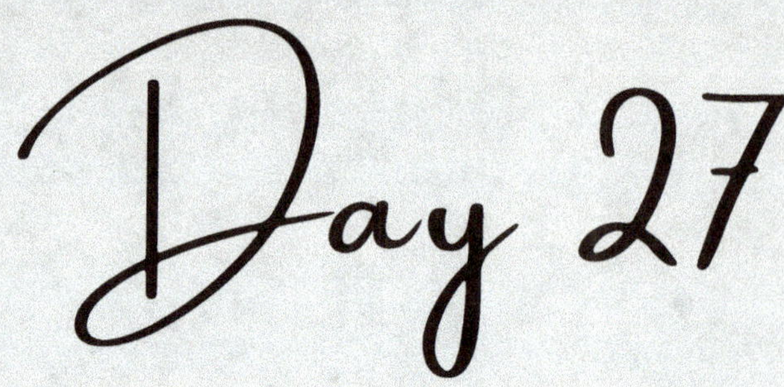

Day 27

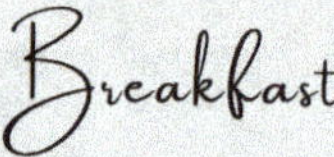

Breakfast

Egg and Veggie Breakfast Muffins
Ingredients:
- Eggs
- Chopped bell peppers
- Diced onions
- Spinach
- Instructions: Whisk eggs in a bowl, then stir in chopped vegetables. Pour mixture into greased muffin tins and bake at 350°F (175°C) for 20-25 minutes, or until set

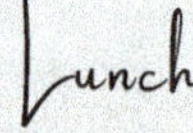

Lunch

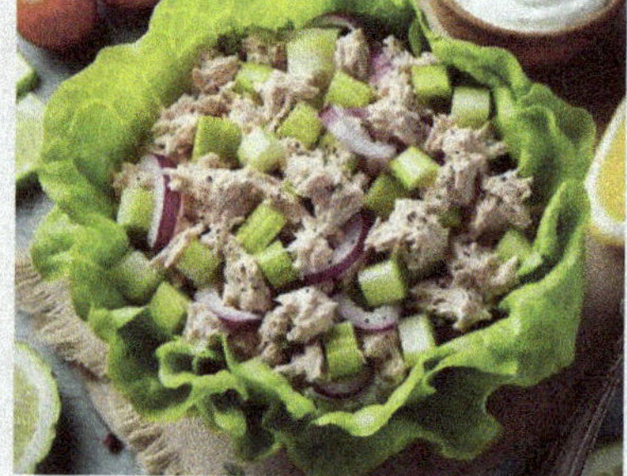

Tuna Salad Lettuce Wraps
Ingredients:
- Canned tuna, drained
- Diced celery
- Diced red onion
- Greek yogurt
- Lettuce leaves
- Instructions: Mix tuna, celery, red onion, and Greek yogurt in a bowl. Spoon onto lettuce leaves and wrap.

Dinner

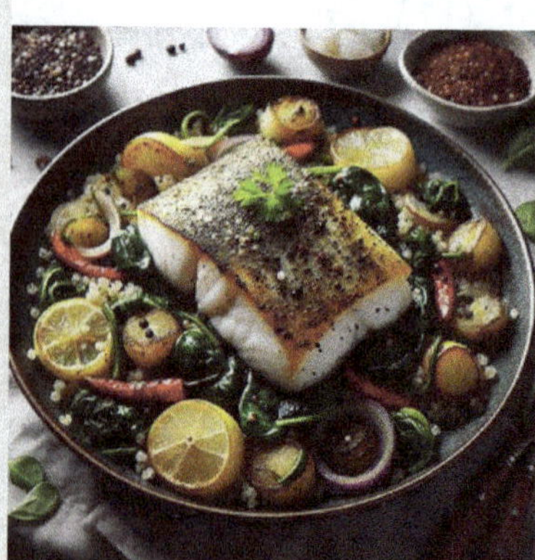

Baked Halibut with Sautéed Spinach and Quinoa
Ingredients:
- Halibut fillets
- spinach
- quinoa
- lemon
- olive oil,
- Garlic powder
- Salt & Pepper
- Instructions: Season halibut fillets with olive oil, lemon juice, minced garlic, salt, and pepper. Bake in the oven at 375°F until cooked through. Sauté spinach with minced garlic in olive oil until wilted. Serve halibut with sautéed spinach and cooked quinoa.

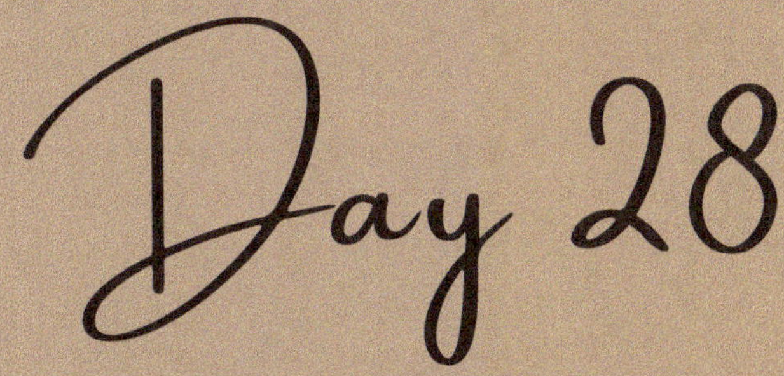

Breakfast

Veggie and Egg Breakfast Burrito
Ingredients:
- Whole wheat tortilla
- Scrambled eggs
- Sautéed bell peppers, onions, and
- spinach
- Salsa (optional)
- Instructions: Fill a whole wheat tortilla with scrambled eggs and sautéed vegetables. Add salsa if desired, then roll up the tortilla to form a burrito.

Lunch

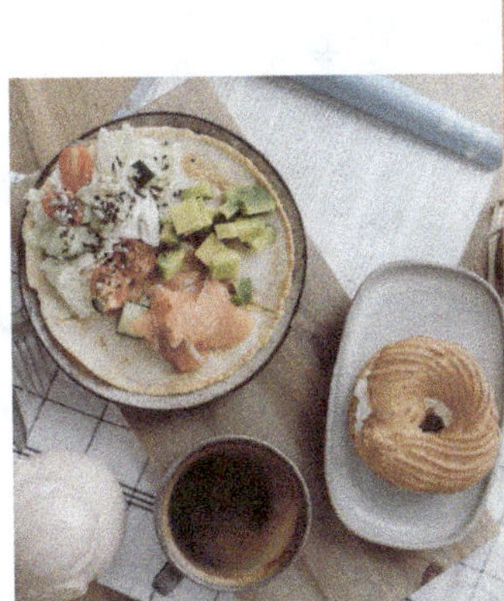

Grilled Salmon Salad with Avocado
Ingredients:
- Grilled salmon fillet
- Mixed greens
- Sliced avocado
- Cherry tomatoes
- Cucumber slices
- Instructions: Arrange all ingredients on a plate and serve with your favorite dressing.

Dinner

Turkey Chili with Beans
Ingredients:
- Ground turkey
- Diced tomatoes
- Kidney beans
- Bell peppers
- Onion
- Chili powder
- Instructions: In a pot, cook ground turkey with diced onions and bell peppers until browned. Add diced tomatoes, kidney beans, and chili powder. Simmer for 30 minutes. Serve hot.

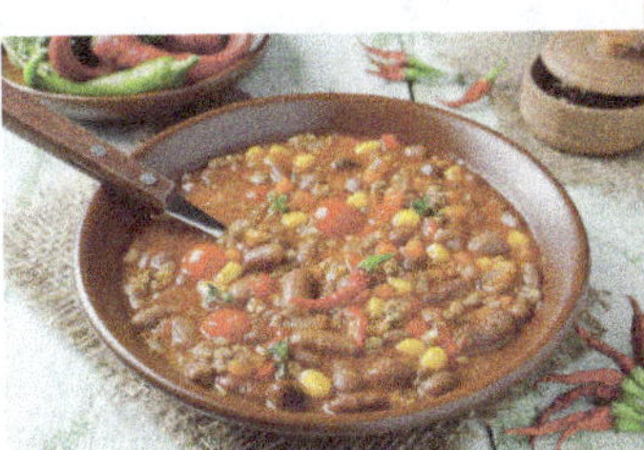

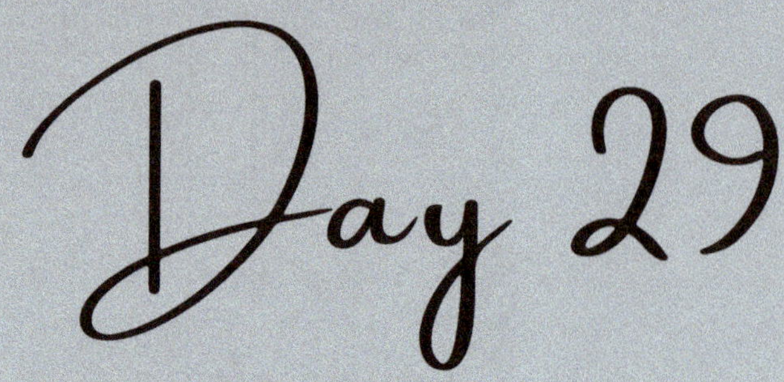

Day 29

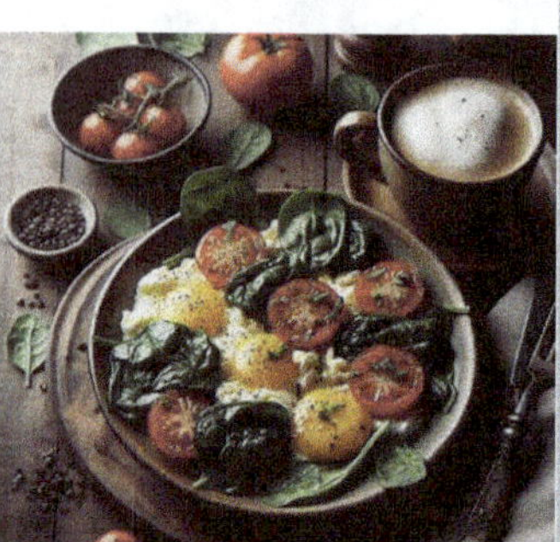

Scrambled Eggs with Spinach and Tomato
Ingredients:

- Eggs
- Handful of spinach
- Diced tomato
- Instructions: Scramble eggs in a pan, then add spinach and diced tomato. Cook until spinach wilts and tomato softens. Season with salt and pepper to taste.

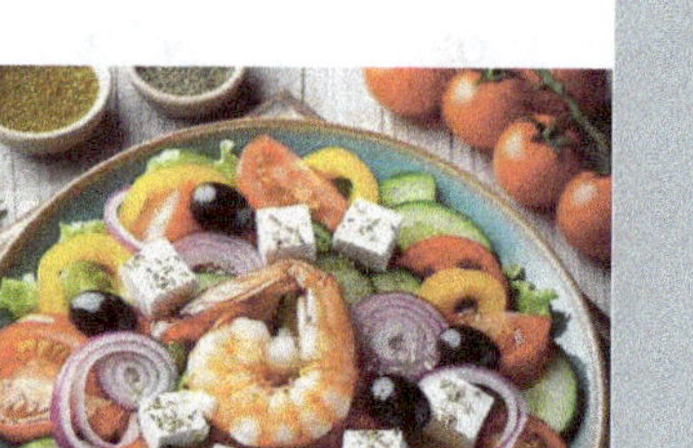

Greek Salad with Grilled Shrimp
Ingredients:

- Mixed greens
- Grilled shrimp
- Diced cucumber, cherry tomatoes, and red onion
- Kalamata olives
- Crumbled feta cheese
- Greek dressing
- Instructions: Toss together all ingredients in a bowl with Greek dressing.

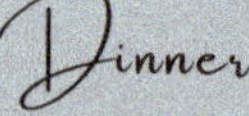

Baked Chicken Thighs with Roasted Carrots and Couscous

- Ingredients:
- Chicken thighs
- Carrots
- Couscous
- Olive oil
- Garlic powder, paprika, salt, pepper
- Instructions: Season chicken thighs with olive oil, garlic powder, paprika, salt, and pepper. Bake in the oven at 400°F until cooked through. Toss carrots with olive oil, salt, and pepper. Roast in the oven until tender. Prepare couscous according to package instructions. Serve chicken thighs with roasted carrots and couscous.

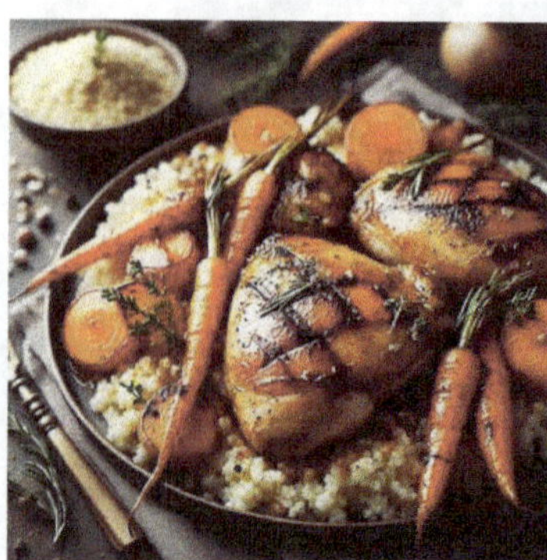

Day 30

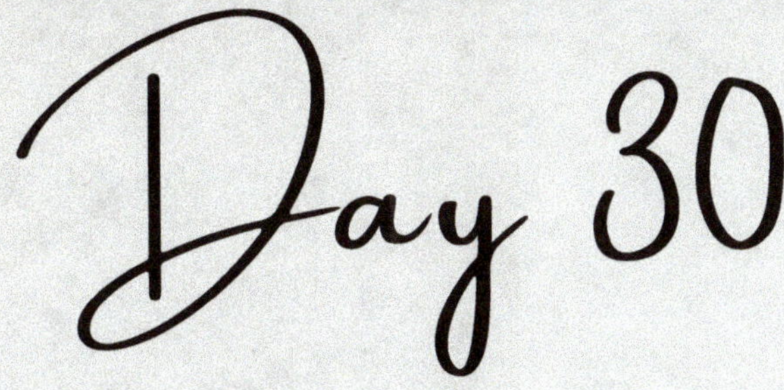

Veggie Omelette with Feta Cheese
Ingredients:

- Eggs
- Diced bell peppers, onions, and tomatoes
- Crumbled feta cheese
- Instructions: Beat eggs in a bowl and pour into a hot skillet. Add diced vegetables and cook until eggs are set. Sprinkle with crumbled feta cheese before serving.

Lunch

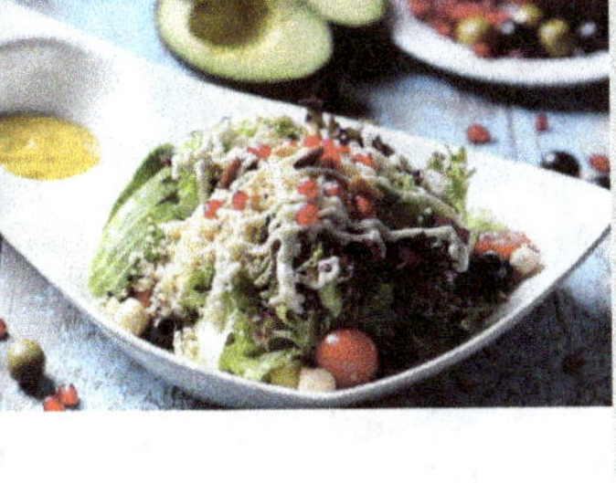

Chicken and Avocado Salad with Cilantro Lime Dressing
Ingredients:

- Grilled chicken breast
- Mixed greens
- Sliced avocado
- Cherry tomatoes
- Cilantro
- Lime juice
- Olive oil
- Salt and pepper to taste
- Instructions: Toss grilled chicken, mixed greens, sliced avocado, and cherry tomatoes in a bowl. In a separate bowl, whisk together chopped cilantro, lime juice, olive oil, salt, and pepper to make the dressing. Drizzle over the salad before serving.

Dinner

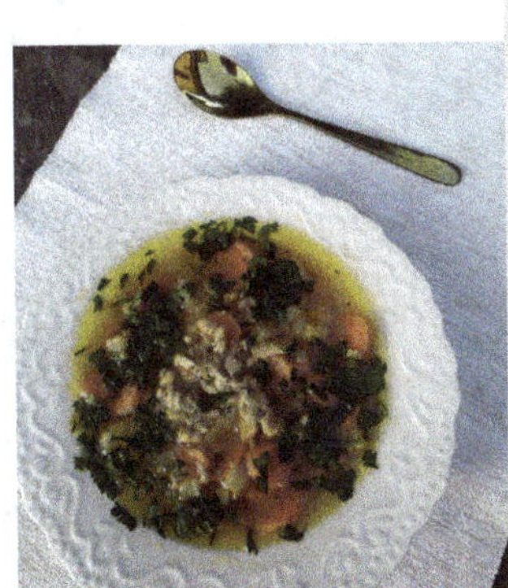

Turkey and Vegetable Soup
Ingredients:

- Ground turkey
- Chopped onions, carrots, and celery
- Diced tomatoes
- Low-sodium chicken broth
- Spinach
- Italian seasoning
- Instructions: In a pot, cook ground turkey with chopped onions, carrots, and celery until turkey is browned. Add diced tomatoes, chicken broth, and Italian seasoning. Simmer for 20-25minutes. Stir in spinach and cook until wilted before serving.

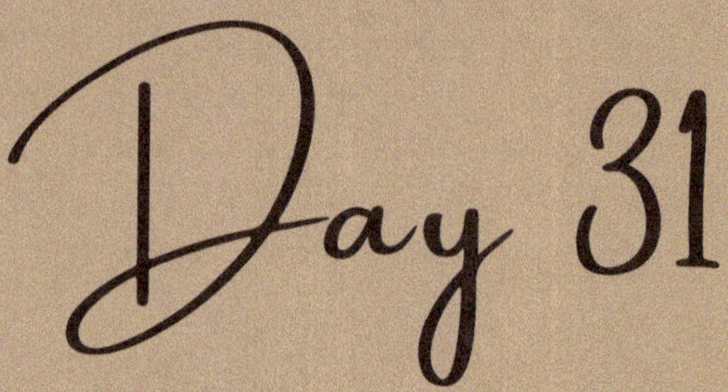

Breakfast

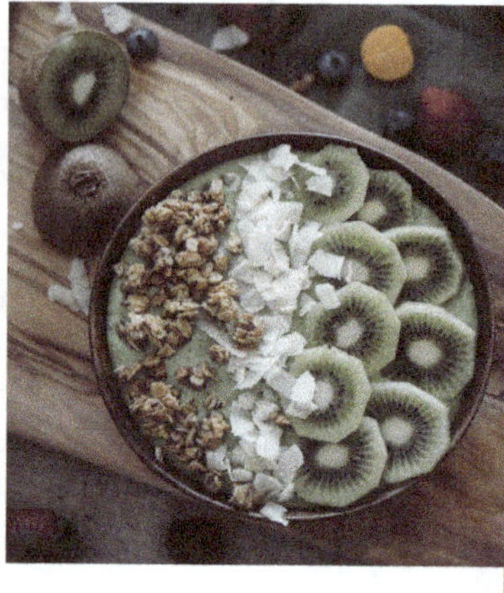

Green Smoothie Bowl with Kiwi and Coconut
Ingredients:
- Handful of spinach
- 1/2 banana
- 1 kiwi, peeled and sliced
- Unsweetened coconut flakes
- Unsweetened almond milk
- Instructions: Blend spinach, banana, kiwi, and almond milk until smooth. Pour into a bowl and top with coconut flakes.

Lunch

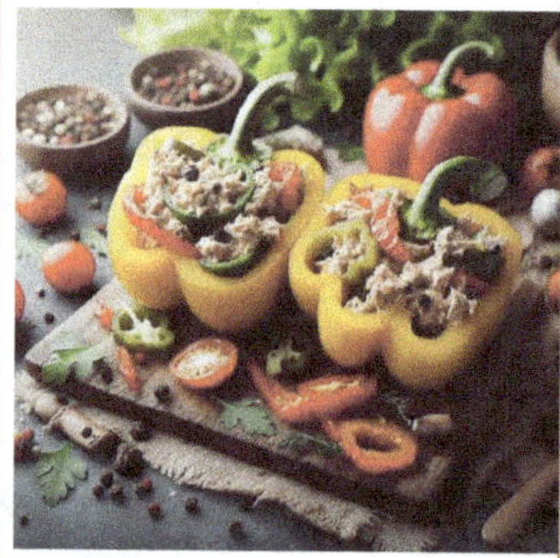

Tuna Salad Stuffed Bell Peppers
Ingredients:
- Canned tuna, drained
- Diced celery and red onion
- Greek yogurt
- Dijon mustard
- Bell peppers, halved and seeds removed
- Instructions: In a bowl, mix tuna, celery, red onion, Greek yogurt, and Dijon mustard. Spoon mixture into halved bell peppers and serve.

Dinner

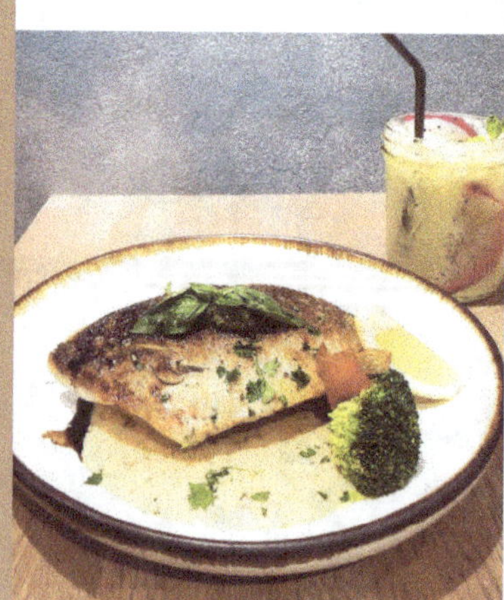

Baked Tilapia with Lemon and Herbs, Served with Steamed Broccoli
Ingredients:
- Tilapia fillets
- Lemon slices
- Fresh herbs (such as parsley, thyme, and
- rosemary)
- Olive oil
- Salt and pepper to taste
- Broccoli florets
- Instructions: Preheat oven to 375°F (190°C). Place tilapia fillets on a baking sheet lined with parchment paper. Top with lemon slices, chopped herbs, olive oil, salt, and pepper. Bake for 12-15 minutes or until fish is cooked through. Serve with steamed broccoli.

Disclaimer

What works for me might not necessarily be your cup of tea. It's always wise to consult your doctor before embarking on any new dietary journey. Feel free to tweak the menu to your heart's content. If a recipe calls for scrambled eggs, but you prefer them sunny side up, go ahead and flip those eggs. Don't hesitate to swap chicken for turkey, or vice versa, if that's more your style. And hey, if you're feeling adventurous, throw in some extra veggies and girl, you can even sprinkle on some additional seasoning until your ancestor's smile. Just remember to keep an eye on that salt intake—no one wants to be caught in a sodium overload!

Burgers for Days

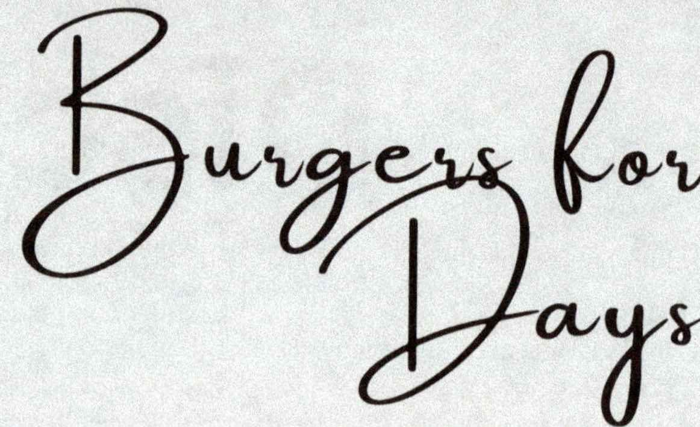

Salmon Burger

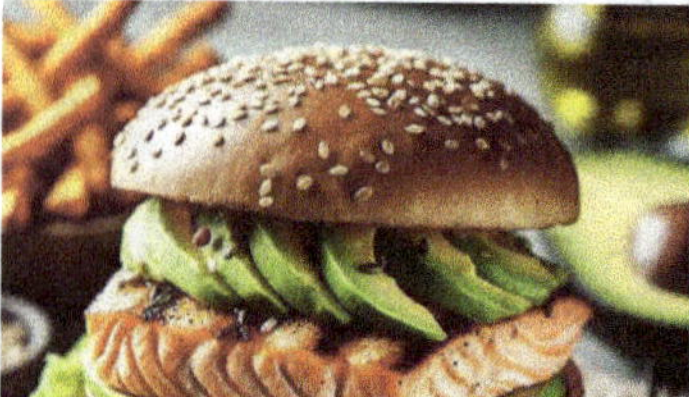

- Preheat grill or skillet over medium heat.
- Season salmon fillets with lemon zest, dill, and Old Bay seasoning.
- Grill salmon fillets for about 4-5 minutes on each side, or until cooked through.
- Toast whole wheat buns if desired.
- Assemble burgers by placing cooked salmon fillets on buns and topping with cucumber slices, red onion, and tzatziki sauce.

Black Bean Sweet Potato Burger

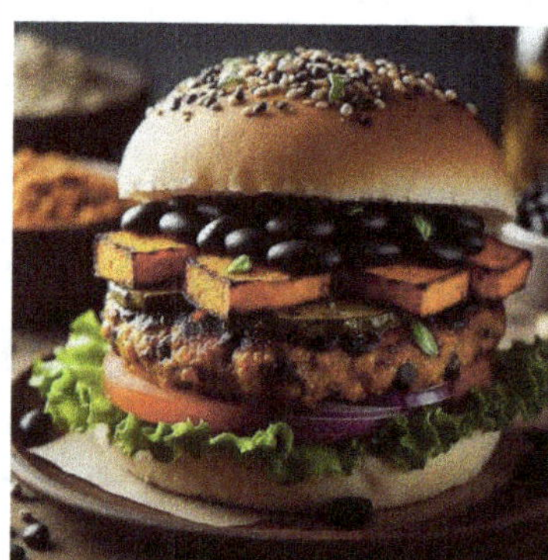

- Preheat oven to 375°F (190°C).
- In a bowl, mash cooked sweet potatoes with cooked black beans, diced red onion, chopped cilantro, cumin, smoked paprika, and a dash of hot sauce.
- Form mixture into patties and place on a baking sheet lined with parchment paper.
- Bake patties for about 25-30 minutes, flipping halfway through, until crispy and heated through.
- Toast whole grain buns if desired.
- Assemble burgers by placing cooked patties on buns and topping with sliced avocado and arugula.

Greek Lamb Burger

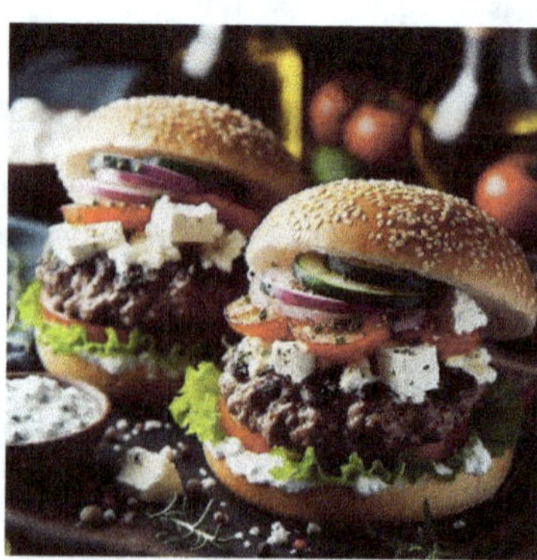

- Preheat grill or skillet over medium heat.
- In a bowl, mix ground lamb with minced garlic, chopped fresh mint, dried oregano, salt, and pepper.
- Form mixture into patties.
- Grill patties for about 4-5 minutes on each side, or until cooked to your desired doneness.
- Toast whole grain buns if desired.
- Assemble burgers by placing cooked patties on buns and topping with crumbled feta cheese, sliced cucumber, red onion, and tzatziki sauce. Optional: Serve with a side of Greek salad or roasted vegetables for a complete meal.

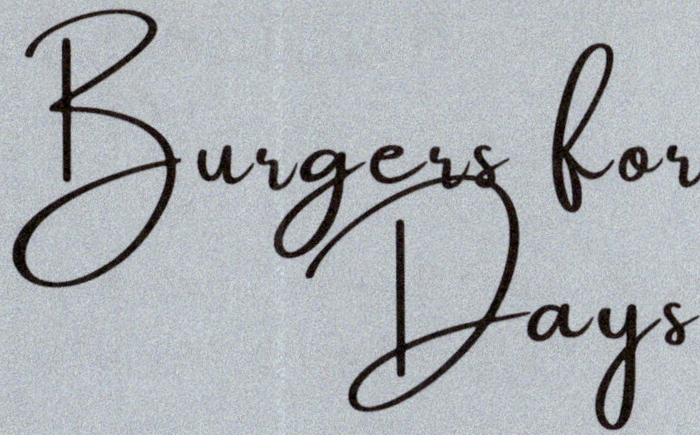

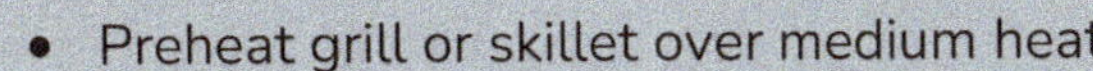

Turkey Avocado Burger:

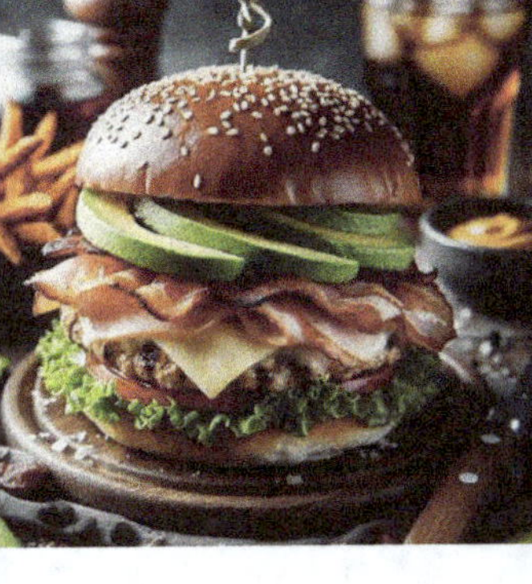

- Preheat grill or skillet over medium heat.
- Mix ground turkey with garlic powder, onion powder, and paprika. Form into patties.
- Cook patties for about 5-6 minutes on each side, or until fully cooked.
- Toast whole grain buns if desired.
- Assemble burgers by placing cooked patties on buns and topping with sliced avocado, tomato, lettuce, and a dollop of Greek yogurt mixed with lime juice and cilantro. Add turkey bacon if desired.

Portobello Mushroom Burger

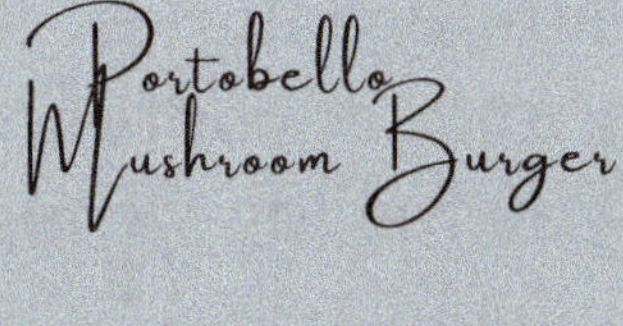

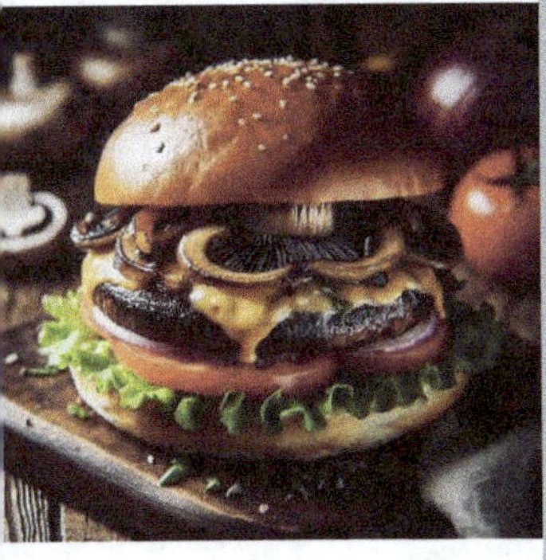

- Preheat grill or skillet over medium heat.
- Marinate portobello mushroom caps in balsamic vinegar, olive oil, and minced garlic for 20-30 minutes.
- Grill mushroom caps for about 4-5 minutes on each side, or until tender.
- Toast whole grain buns if desired.
- Assemble burgers by placing grilled mushroom caps on buns and topping with roasted red peppers, spinach, and melted mozzarella cheese.

Quinoa Veggie Burger

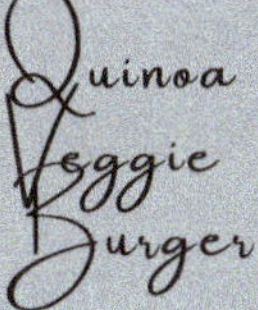

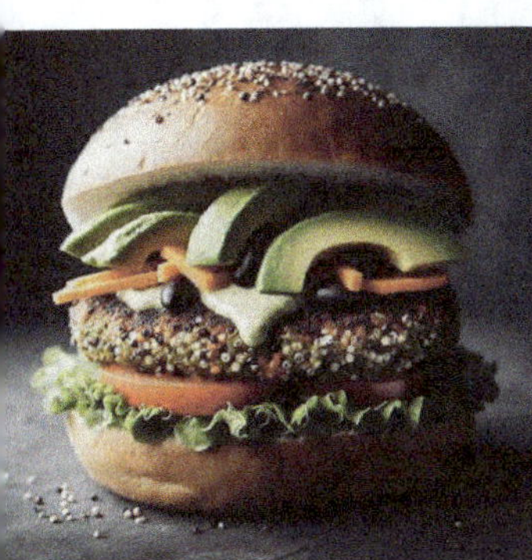

- Preheat grill or skillet over medium heat.
- In a bowl, mix cooked quinoa with grated carrots, chopped bell peppers, black beans, breadcrumbs, cumin, chili powder, and garlic powder.
- Form mixture into patties.
- Grill patties for about 4-5 minutes on each side, or until golden brown and heated through.
- Toast whole grain buns if desired.
- Assemble burgers by placing cooked patties on buns and topping with lettuce, tomato, and avocado slices.

Nutritional Information Guide

Alright, sis, let's talk about how to read those nutrition labels and make smart choice about what we're putting on our plates. Here's the lowdown to help you navigate thos labels like a boss:

- **Serving Sizes:** Pay attention to the serving size listed on the label – that's the amount of food they consider one serving. Keep it real and be mindful of portion sizes to avoid overdoing it.
- **Calories:** Check out how many calories are in each serving. That tells you how much energy you're getting from the food. If you're trying to shed a few pounds, opt for foods with fewer calories, but remember, it's not just about the numbers – go for nutrient-rich foods over empty calories.
- **Macronutrients:** Look at the protein, carbs, and fat content per serving. Aim for a good balance of these nutrients to keep you feeling strong and satisfied.
- **Fiber:** Girl, we love fiber! It helps keep us full and keeps things moving, if you know what I mean. Look for foods with plenty of fiber – shoot for at least 3 grams per serving.
- **Sugars:** Keep an eye out for added sugars in processed foods. Choose options with less sugar or go for natural sweetness like fruit.
- **Sodium:** Watch that sodium content, especially if you're trying to keep that bloat in check or keep your blood pressure in check. Opt for lower-sodium options when you can.
- **Ingredients List:** Take a peek at the ingredients list to see what's really in there. Stick to products with fewer ingredients and steer clear of added preservatives, artificial colors, and flavors.

Remember, queen, it's all about focusing on whole, real foods and keeping an eye on those portion sizes. By understanding those labels, you can make choices that'll keep you feeling fierce and on track with your health goals. You got this!

Ingredient Substitution: So, you won't jump to Conclusions.

Here's an example of ingredient substitutions to help you out in a pinch or accommodate dietary needs:

- **Buttermilk:** Substitute 1 cup of buttermilk with 1 tablespoon of lemon juice or white vinegar plus enough milk to make 1 cup. Let it sit for 5-10 minutes before using.
- **Eggs (for binding):** Substitute 1 egg with 1/4 cup of unsweetened applesauce, mashed banana, or plain yogurt.
- **All-Purpose Flour:** Substitute 1 cup of all-purpose flour with 1 cup of whole wheat flour or 1/2 cup of almond flour plus 1/2 cup of coconut flour for gluten-free options.
- **White Sugar:** Substitute 1 cup of white sugar with 3/4 cup of honey or maple syrup, or 1 cup of mashed bananas or unsweetened applesauce for a healthier alternative.
- **Butter:** Substitute 1 cup of butter with 1 cup of coconut oil or 1 cup of Greek yogurt for baking, or 1 cup of mashed avocado for spreading on toast or sandwiches.
- **Heavy Cream:** Substitute 1 cup of heavy cream with 1 cup of coconut cream or full-fat coconut milk, or 1 cup of Greek yogurt thinned with a little water.
- **Breadcrumbs:** Substitute 1 cup of breadcrumbs with 1 cup of crushed cornflakes, rolled oats, or crushed crackers.
- **Soy Sauce:** Substitute 1 tablespoon of soy sauce with 1 tablespoon of tamari sauce for a gluten-free option, or 1 tablespoon of coconut aminos for a soy-free option.
- **Parmesan Cheese:** Substitute 1/4 cup of Parmesan cheese with 1/4 cup of nutritional yeast for a vegan alternative, or 1/4 cup of grated pecorino Romano cheese for a sharper flavor.
- **Vegetable Oil:** Substitute 1 cup of vegetable oil with 1 cup of melted coconut oil, olive oil, or avocado oil, depending on the recipe.

Conversion Charts for your Shopping Carts

Cooking can be a science, but don't worry, I've got you covered with these handy conversion charts to help you navigate your way around the kitchen like a pro:

Measurement Conversions:

- 1 teaspoon (tsp) = 5 milliliters (ml)
- 1 tablespoon (tbsp) = 15 milliliters (ml)
- 1 fluid ounce (fl oz) = 29.5735 milliliters (ml)
- 1 cup = 8 fluid ounces = 236.588 milliliters (ml) 1 pint = 2 cups = 16 fluid ounces = 473.176 milliliters (ml)
- 1 quart = 4 cups = 32 fluid ounces = 946.353 milliliters (ml)
- 1 gallon = 4 quarts = 128 fluid ounces = 3.78541 liters (L)

Liquid Measurements:

- 1 milliliter (ml) = 0.033814 fluid ounces (fl oz)
- 1 liter (L) = 1000 milliliters (ml) = 33.814 fluid ounces (fl oz)
- 1 fluid ounce (fl oz) = 29.5735 milliliters (ml)
- 1 cup = 8 fluid ounces = 236.588 milliliters (ml) 1 pint = 16 fluid ounces = 473.176 milliliters (ml)
- 1 quart = 32 fluid ounces = 946.353 milliliters (ml)
- 1 gallon = 128 fluid ounces = 3.78541 liters (L)

Weight Conversions:

- 1 ounce (oz) = 28.3495 grams (g)
- 1 pound (lb) = 16 ounces (oz) = 453.592 grams (g)
- 1 gram (g) = 0.035274 ounces (oz)
- 1 kilogram (kg) = 1000 grams (g) = 35.274 ounces (oz) = 2.20462 pounds (lb)

Common Cooking Units:

- 1 stick of butter = ½ cup = 8 tablespoons = 113 grams
- 1 cup of flour = 120 grams
- 1 cup of sugar = 200 grams
- 1 cup of oats = 90 grams
- 1 cup of rice = 200 grams (uncooked)

These conversion charts will make it a breeze to follow recipes from around the world and ensure your culinary creations turn out just right every time. Happy cooking!

Cheat Sheet

Check it out, sis! These are my top-secret cheat codes for hacking your progress and making those pounds disappear like magic! Trust me, I've put these tactics to the test, and the results? They speak for themselves!

Steer clear of buying cooking grease, not only to save some cash but also to encourage yourself to explore innovative cooking methods that are healthier and more exciting! If you're absolutely itching for fried foods and just are in dire need, try out these strategies:

- Opt for dining out at restaurants to avoid the temptation of using excessive grease in your meals when cooking at home later.
- Share your purchases with someone to resist the temptations of eating everything by yourself. If you have boys in the house like me, they love leftovers. (If they didn't join you for dinner)
- Where I saw major results. Instead of indulging in those wings and fries, break the wings up and incorporate them into a garden salad. If you have to have the fries eat six to satisfy the urge.
- Bread off, flavor on! Unleash the true essence of your burger without the bun. Or have a Flying Dutchman burger and use onions for the bun instead.
- Eat high and low-metabolism foods together. So, if you have a slice of pizza (low metabolism) eat it with an apple (high metabolism)

Skip sugary drinks altogether. Since I'm not much of a breakfast person, I opted for a homemade smoothie with fruits and vegetables to ensure I didn't miss any meals. You can also:

- Drink water infused with fruit slices.
- Unsweetened herbal tea or green tea
- Sparkling water with a splash of lemon or lime juice
- Plain black coffee or espresso
- Vegetable juice

When indulging in a salad, it's essential to ensure it stays healthy. Here are several tips to help you maintain its nutritional value and make it a nourishing meal:

- Load up your salad with fresh veggies, lean proteins, and healthy fats.
- Use homemade dressings with olive oil and vinegar instead of store-bought ones.
- Keep portion sizes in check and avoid high-calorie toppings.
- Instead of eating whole croutons, crunch up about five and sprinkle them over your salad. thank me later.
- Take a regular serving size of dressing, add it to your salad in a container with a lid, then shake it up to evenly coat all of your salad.
- Keep in mind the healthy dressing serving sizes; 1 salad = 2 TBSP of creamy dressing, 1.5 TBSP of vinegarette, and if it's the main course 2.5 TBSP per person.

Incorporating these three straightforward steps into your routine ensures that your journey toward a healthier diet will be not only successful but also enjoyable. With mindful choices in ingredients, portion control, and preparation techniques, you'll be well-equipped to achieve your wellness goals while savoring every bite along the way.

Cheat Sheet

When snack cravings hit between meals, I raided the pantry like a snack-hungry ninja. From celery sticks begging for peanut butter love to pizza slices that vanished faster than my willpower, my snack adventures were a comedy of cravings.

When the snack attack started to hit me, here is a list of items I snacked on in between meals that are budget-friendly.

Fruits with Protein:

- Apple slices with almond butter
- Banana with peanut butter
- Orange segments with Greek yogurt
- Berries (strawberries, blueberries, raspberries) with cottage cheese
- Grapes with cheese cubes
- Pineapple chunks with turkey slices
- Watermelon cubes with sliced almonds
- Kiwi slices with Greek yogurt
- Mango chunks with cottage cheese
- Pear slices with almond butter

Crackers and Chips with Spreads:

- Rice cakes with avocado
- Whole grain crackers with cheese slices
- Rice crackers with hummus
- Tortilla chips with guacamole
- Pita chips with tzatziki
- Multigrain crackers with cream cheese
- Pretzel sticks with peanut butter
- Veggie chips with Greek yogurt dip
- Popcorn with melted dark chocolate
- Seaweed snacks with sesame seed hummus

Vegetables with Dips:

- Baby carrots with hummus
- Cucumber slices with tzatziki
- Cherry tomatoes with Greek yogurt dip
- Bell pepper strips with ranch dip
- Snap peas with hummus
- Celery sticks with peanut butter
- Broccoli florets with Greek yogurt dip
- Cauliflower florets with hummus
- Radish slices with tzatziki
- Zucchini sticks with marinara sauce

Nuts and Seeds with Fruits:

- Almonds with apple slices
- Walnuts with banana slices
- Cashews with orange segments
- Pistachios with grapes
- Pumpkin seeds with pineapple chunks
- Sunflower seeds with kiwi slices
- Hazelnuts with mango chunks
- Pecans with pear slices
- Chia seeds with mixed berries
- Flaxseeds with watermelon cubes

Jerky and Protein Bars with Miscellaneous:

- Beef jerky with popcorn
- Turkey jerky with rice cakes
- Protein bar with nuts
- Chicken jerky with rice crackers
- Salmon jerky with veggie chips
- Tofu jerky with dried fruit
- Bison jerky with granola bars
- Pork jerky with rice chips
- Veggie jerky with dark chocolate squares
- Bean jerky with seaweed snacks

These snacks are just a sample of healthy, low-calorie options that can help you feel satisfied and energized throughout the day.

Notes

Notes

THANK YOU

DEAR BEAUTIFUL SOULS,

AS I SIT DOWN TO WRITE THIS, I'M OVERWHELMED WITH GRATITUDE FOR EACH AND EVERY ONE OF YOU WHO HAS JOINED ME ON THIS INCREDIBLE JOURNEY. FROM THE DEPTHS OF MY HEART, THANK YOU FOR CHOOSING TO EMBARK ON THIS TRANSFORMATIVE ADVENTURE TOWARD HEALTH AND WELLNESS ALONGSIDE ME.

FIRST AND FOREMOST, I WANT TO EXPRESS MY DEEPEST APPRECIATION TO THE INCREDIBLE COMMUNITY OF BLACK WOMEN WHO HAVE INSPIRED AND MOTIVATED ME EVERY STEP OF THE WAY. YOUR STRENGTH, RESILIENCE, AND UNWAVERING SUPPORT HAVE BEEN THE DRIVING FORCE BEHIND THIS PROJECT, AND I AM FOREVER GRATEFUL FOR YOUR LOVE AND ENCOURAGEMENT.

TO MY AMAZING READERS, THANK YOU FOR ENTRUSTING ME WITH YOUR HEALTH AND WELL-BEING. YOUR WILLINGNESS TO EMBRACE CHANGE AND COMMIT TO MAKING POSITIVE LIFESTYLE SHIFTS FILLS ME WITH IMMENSE PRIDE AND JOY. REMEMBER, YOU ARE CAPABLE OF ACHIEVING ANYTHING YOU SET YOUR MIND TO, AND I AM HERE TO CHEER YOU ON EVERY STEP OF THE WAY.

I AM INDEBTED TO THE COUNTLESS INDIVIDUALS WHO CONTRIBUTED THEIR TIME, EXPERTISE, AND WISDOM TO THE CREATION OF THIS BOOK. FROM NUTRITIONISTS AND FITNESS EXPERTS TO CHEFS AND WELLNESS COACHES, YOUR INSIGHTS HAVE BEEN INVALUABLE IN SHAPING THE CONTENT AND ENSURING ITS ACCURACY AND RELEVANCE.

A SPECIAL SHOUTOUT GOES TO MY FAMILY, FRIENDS, AND LOVED ONES FOR THEIR UNWAVERING SUPPORT AND ENCOURAGEMENT THROUGHOUT THIS JOURNEY. YOUR BELIEF IN ME AND YOUR ENDLESS WORDS OF ENCOURAGEMENT HAVE KEPT ME GOING THROUGH THE UPS AND DOWNS, AND I AM ETERNALLY GRATEFUL FOR YOUR LOVE AND ENCOURAGEMENT.

LAST BUT CERTAINLY NOT LEAST, I WANT TO EXPRESS MY DEEPEST GRATITUDE TO THE ANCESTORS AND TRAILBLAZERS WHO PAVED THE WAY FOR US TO THRIVE AND FLOURISH. YOUR RESILIENCE, STRENGTH, AND UNWAVERING SPIRIT CONTINUE TO INSPIRE US TO REACH FOR THE STARS AND LIVE OUR BEST LIVES.

IN CLOSING, I WANT TO EXTEND MY HEARTFELT THANKS TO EACH AND EVERY ONE OF YOU FOR YOUR LOVE, SUPPORT, AND COMMITMENT TO YOUR HEALTH AND WELL-BEING. REMEMBER, YOU ARE CAPABLE OF ACHIEVING ANYTHING YOU SET YOUR MIND TO, AND I AM HONORED TO BE A PART OF YOUR JOURNEY TOWARD A HEALTHIER, HAPPIER YOU.

WITH LOVE AND GRATITUDE,

D.K.R.G

"IF YOU CAN'T FLY, THEN RUN, IF YOU CAN'T WALK RUN, THEN WALK, IF YOU CAN'T WALK, THEN CRAWL, BUT BY ALL MEANS KEEP MOVING." –

MARTIN LUTHER KING JR.